Avoiding Burnout

Avoiding Burnout

*How Exemplary Teachers
Find Fuel and Cultivate Success*

Betsy B. Nordell

ROWMAN & LITTLEFIELD
Lanham • Boulder • New York • London

Published by Rowman & Littlefield
An imprint of The Rowman & Littlefield Publishing Group, Inc.
4501 Forbes Boulevard, Suite 200, Lanham, Maryland 20706
www.rowman.com

6 Tinworth Street, London SE11 5AL, United Kingdom

Copyright © 2021 by Betsy B. Nordell

All rights reserved. No part of this book may be reproduced in any form or by any electronic or mechanical means, including information storage and retrieval systems, without written permission from the publisher, except by a reviewer who may quote passages in a review.

British Library Cataloguing in Publication Information Available

Library of Congress Cataloging-in-Publication Data

Names: Nordell, Betsy B., 1963– author.
Title: Avoiding burnout : how exemplary teachers find fuel and cultivate success / Betsy B. Nordell.
Description: Lanham : Rowman & Littlefield, [2021] | Includes bibliographical references and index. | Summary: "The book is specifically designed to spur thinking and conversation about what supports and inhibits educator success"— Provided by publisher.
Identifiers: LCCN 2020011070 (print) | LCCN 2020011071 (ebook) | ISBN 9781475855241 (cloth) | ISBN 9781475855258 (paperback) | ISBN 9781475855265 (epub)
Subjects: LCSH: Teachers—Job stress. | Burn out (Psychology) | Teacher effectiveness. | Mindfulness (Psychology)
Classification: LCC LB2840.2 .N67 2020 (print) | LCC LB2840.2 (ebook) | DDC 371.1001/9—dc23
LC record available at https://lccn.loc.gov/2020011070
LC ebook record available at https://lccn.loc.gov/2020011071

∞ ™ The paper used in this publication meets the minimum requirements of American National Standard for Information Sciences Permanence of Paper for Printed Library Materials, ANSI/NISO Z39.48-1992.

To John, Meredith, and Andrew.

Contents

Acknowledgments — ix

Introduction — xi

I: How Teachers See Their Work — 1
1. Teacher Power — 5
2. The Gift of Providing a Fresh Start — 13
3. Meaning and Purpose — 23

II: The Central Role of Relationships — 33
4. Knowing Students Well — 37
5. Cultivating Positive Relationships With Students — 45
6. Negotiating Difficult Relationships With Students — 57
7. Investing in a Positive Learning Environment — 67
8. Connecting With Parents and Caregivers — 77
9. Relationships With Colleagues — 85
10. The Administration of Schools — 101

III: Personal Practices and Skills — 115
11. Curiosity — 117
12. Reflection — 127
13. Preparation and Self-Care — 139

14 What Makes Great Teachers Great?	153
Appendixes	159
Appendix A: The Tale of the Stonecutters	161
Appendix B: Knowing My Students	163
Appendix C: Staff Directory of Support	165
Appendix D: Standpoint Exploration	167
Appendix E: Exploring Hope	169
Appendix F: Free Resources and Additional Materials	175
Notes	179
References	197
Index	209
About the Author	215

Acknowledgments

Avoiding Burnout: How Exemplary Teachers Find Fuel and Cultivate Success would not be possible without the generosity of the exemplary teachers who agreed to participate in my study. It was an honor to spend time with them. They are brilliant educators and inspiring human beings.

Throughout the long process of writing this book, I benefited greatly from the efforts of many at Wellesley College. First, the Wellesley College library staff provided easy access to an extraordinary array of compelling and helpful resources. Layli Maparyan's leadership of the Wellesley Centers for Women (WCW) created two pivotal opportunities that shaped the book's content: S.E.E.D. (Seeking Educational Equity and Diversity) training and the WCW Writing Group. I extend many thanks to Layli, my S.E.E.D. trainers—Karen Lachance, Kamilah Drummond-Forrester, Emmy Howe, Emily Style—and my WCW Writing Group colleagues.

Experiences with current Open Circle staff members—Kamilah Drummond-Forrester, Nancy MacKay, Sallie Dunning, Peg Sawyer, Jen Dirga, Mary Frederick, Christina Wong Chin, Sheila McManus—along with past Open Circle colleagues since 1993, have deepened my thinking about schools and teaching. A special thanks also goes to Leading Together's Pamela Seigle and Chip Wood, education innovators and inspiring models of curiosity, openness, and leadership.

I have been fortunate to have taught and coached administrators and teachers with Open Circle and Leading Together. Time spent with these educators enhanced my understanding and galvanized my desire to create work to address their well-being.

I owe a great debt to my teachers—Tal Ben-Shahar, Ellen Langer, Daniel Goleman, Ryan Niemiec, Robert Biswas-Diener, Bruce Wellman, Nadine Bonda, Paula Green—who have helped me see the world in a significantly different way. I also want to appreciate the thought-provoking and influential writing of Peter Senge, Otto Scharmer, Jennifer Eberhardt, Barbara Fredrickson, Susan Smalley, Diana Winston, Kerry Howells, Margaret Cullen, Adam Grant, Amy Wrzesniewski, Parker Palmer, David Cooperrider, Angela Bahns, Doris Santoro, and the late Shane Lopez.

I want to also extend my warm appreciation to others who have influenced my journey with this book. For so many years, conversations with the knowledgeable and curious Cathy Pastan, Steven Levy, Meenakshi Chhabra, and Linda Ayer have enhanced my life. At the end of every conversation with each of them, I have felt empowered and enriched.

The online Relational-Cultural Theory antiracism working group, spearheaded by Harriet Schwartz, expanded my awareness and thinking. More recently, Harriet also provided helpful feedback on Chapter 12. Much of the content included in Chapter 14 arose as an answer to the question "What's your acronym?" posed by my friend, the thoughtful and inquisitive educator Linda Hall. Steadfast early supporters Mary Duncan, Meredith Shaw, Elizabeth Oriel, Melissa Urey, Laura Thomas, Susan Dreyer-Leon, and Joy Kaubin helped get me started with this work.

Christine Michael, Judith Klimkiewicz, Lynne Celli, and Nick Young nurtured the ideas that led to the research that served as the basis of this book. The well-connected and generous Mary McClintock directed me to two people who helped refine the book's overall content: Laurie Gullion and Karen Warren. Their direct and clear feedback has helped shape what the book has become. I appreciate Tom Koerner, Carlie Wall, and others at Rowman and Littlefield who believed in the book and supported its creation.

I close this acknowledgment with an expression of thanks to my family for their interest and support over the years—Joe, Brenda, Eric, Anne, Elizabeth, Rudy, Ella, Popo, Joan, and, of course, dear Rodrigo. Last, and in no way least, I feel deep gratitude for John, Meredith, and Andrew—thank you all!

Introduction

Teaching is a complex profession. A variety of factors influence teacher dissatisfaction and stress, such as having too much to teach in too little time, with a classroom of students who have a diverse set of learning needs, in an educational environment influenced by ongoing standardized testing. Burnout and teacher turnover are common.[1] I am passionate about the field of teacher and administrator well-being and want to find ways to support educators so they are better able to bring the best of what they have to offer to their significant and essential work.

Throughout my more than 25 years in teacher education, one topic has particularly captured my interest. It is encapsulated in Parker Palmer's idea that "we teach who we are."[2] The implications and possibilities associated with that statement intrigued me when I was a classroom teacher, and the idea continues to ground my work. In fact, the desire to learn more about *who great teachers are* served as the core of my 2017 doctoral research project that inspired this book.

Given the challenges facing teachers today, I think it is vital that we better understand the workings of educator excellence beyond subject-matter knowledge (*the what*) and applied teaching techniques (*the how*). Who are the educators who exceed the state standards set for teacher performance? What do they do that yields such positive educational outcomes? Are they truly exceptional human beings, so their results cannot easily be generalized to others? Or are there aspects of what they know, think, believe, and do that, if better understood, could be adapted for use by others? Exploring possible answers to those questions concerning teaching excellence serves as the basis of *Avoiding Burnout: How Exemplary Teachers Find Fuel and Cultivate Success*.

ORIGINS OF MY RESEARCH

My curiosity about great teachers was piqued during my Master of Education program. I had the good fortune of getting to know two inspiring educators in the course of my practicums, and they have had a significant influence on the educator I have become.

My first student-teacher placement was right across the hall from Bobbi Fisher, author of *Joyful Learning in Kindergarten*.[3] During that practicum, I would often arrive very early to school in order to spend time with Bobbi while she set up her materials for the day. Bobbi had an infectious enthusiasm for the teaching profession. She was extremely generous and helpful during our early-morning conversations about how to organize and run a classroom. Her comments helped me appreciate the science and art of teaching.

A few months later, I was placed as a student teacher in Steven Levy's classroom. He wrote *Starting From Scratch: One Classroom Builds Its Own Curriculum*.[4] Steven's thoughtfulness and intentionality as an educator informed my foundational beliefs about what it means to be a teacher, for he can hold the big picture and small details that support effective teaching and deep, authentic learning. I learned even more when Steven and I went on to share a fourth-grade classroom as colleagues. Both Bobbi and Steven greatly affected my development and sparked my ongoing interest in educator excellence (K–16).

I invite you to think about your own development as an educator.

- Who has positively influenced you in the past? In what ways did they affect your foundational beliefs about teaching and learning? What are some of the key lessons you learned from them?
- Who do you find inspiring now?

DEFINING *GREAT*

When you think about the words *great teacher*, what comes to mind? One of the biggest challenges of my research was to figure out what *great teaching* means. I considered various standards. Ultimately, being rated "exemplary" overall for at least one year using Massachusetts's teacher-assessment rubrics served as the criteria for inclusion in the project.

The small population of teachers who earn an "exemplary" rating represent the most skillful of all educators in the state. Importantly, Massachusetts public schools routinely receive some of the highest national educational rankings.[5] Therefore, the educators included in the study are some of the most distinguished teachers in the United States.

For those unfamiliar with the teacher-evaluation system in Massachusetts, an "exemplary" rating is the highest possible designation, followed by "proficient," "needs improvement," and "unsatisfactory." In 2015–2016, when 67,572 Massachusetts teachers (K–12) were evaluated, 10.7% were rated "exemplary," 84.7% were rated "proficient," 4.1% were rated "needs improvement," and .4% were rated "unsatisfactory."[6] The Massachusetts Department of Education definition of *exemplary* is

> The educator's performance consistently and significantly exceeds the requirements. . . . The exemplary level represents the highest level of performance. It exceeds the already high standard of Proficient. A rating of Exemplary is reserved for performance . . . that is of such a high level that it could serve as a model for educators in the school, district, or state."[7]

The Massachusetts Department of Education performance ratings are "based on multiple categories of evidence, including evaluator judgments based on observations and artifacts of professional practice; evidence of fulfillment of both professional practice and student learning goals; and multiple measures of student learning, growth, and achievement."[8]

ABOUT THE STUDY

I used qualitative research methods to uncover the exemplary educators' perceptions about what influences their success. Qualitative inquiry is especially helpful when researching an unclear phenomenon because the methodology seeks to describe, explore, and explain what is poorly understood.[9] It intentionally uses a small, nonrandom group of research participants to discover what is distinctive about the group.[10] Research interviews serve as a vehicle to gain insight into an individual's or a nonrandom group's understanding of experience.[11]

Guest, Bunce, and Johnson conducted a study designed to create a practical guideline for conducting qualitative inquiries so researchers could better budget and plan projects. Their research yielded a general recommendation of 12 participants.[12] Given the nature of qualitative inquiry, there continues to be various recommendations concerning how many participants to include in a study. My study included 13 K–5 Massachusetts exemplary educators from six schools and three districts. Not all Massachusetts districts were contacted about the project. Larger Massachusetts districts were avoided because they tend to be inundated with requests, and many have ongoing research projects that are well established.

For those interested in information about the districts where my study participants taught, Table 1 includes approximations for total district student populations as well as percentages for the free and reduced lunch figures. The latter percentages refer to the percentage of students who receive food subsidies as a result of their families' economic challenges.

Table 1. District Information

District	Student Population	Percentage of Free and Reduced Lunch
1	7,000–7,500	45–50%
2	5,500–6,000	35–40%
3	2,500–3,000	35–40%

In all cases, the research participant recruitment process started with the district's school superintendent. After garnering superintendent approval, I was free to contact each school principal. If the principal approved the research, I was provided with the exemplary practitioners' contact information.

The three most common reasons superintendents and principals gave for not moving forward with the research were (1) they did not want to ask people to do "one more thing," given the highly stressful school climate; (2) they already had research being conducted in the district and/or school; and (3) they did not have anyone who fit the "exemplary teacher" criteria. The exemplary educators who declined to participate in the research typically referenced a lack of time as their reason for not becoming involved, although most wished me well with the project.

It took 9 months, 68 district superintendent letters, 55 principal letters, and 22 teacher contacts to find the 13 teachers from 6 schools who ultimately participated in my study. They range in age from 28 to 65 years and have from 6 to 33 years of classroom teaching experience. All self-identified as female and White. I, too, identify as female and White. It is necessary to highlight that the unintentional homogeneity of the research subjects in concert with my background informs and affects the research outcomes. Hearing the perspectives of exemplary educators who do not identify as female and White would have added tremendous value.

When I designed this research, I did not set out to study only White women educators. Being a Massachusetts K–5 teacher who earned an "exemplary" overall rating for at least one year was the criteria. Gender identification, ethnicity, and cultural background are foundational aspects of identity, influencing the way we each make sense of and move through the world. At the time of the study and the publication of this book, information regarding the ethnicity, cultural background, and gender of the overall population of K–5 Massachusetts teachers rated "exemplary" overall was not available.

A forthcoming first-of-its-kind publication, *Handbook of Research on Teachers of Color*, coedited by University of Houston's Conra Gist and University of California, Berkeley's Travis Bristol, will provide concrete practices, rigorous research findings, and helpful information designed to foster rich discussion about teacher diversity. For further details about this publication and additional related links, please see *Experiences of Teachers of Color* in Appendix F.

Each exemplary educator interview occurred once and lasted 63 minutes on average. The teachers' voices heavily populate the text of this book. I found hearing the teachers describe how they negotiate their challenges and cultivate success to be particularly powerful, so I wanted you to have the chance to hear directly from the educators themselves. To protect anonymity, a pseudonym identifies each educator. The name selected reflects the teacher's ethnicity and self-identified cultural background but does not reflect the educator's real name. Table 2 uses a numerical system to share more information about the participating educators without compromising their anonymity.

Table 2. Study Participant Demographics

	Age	Total Years Teaching	Total Years - Current Grade	Total Years - Current School	Highest Degree
Teacher 1	52	18	1	17	Master's
Teacher 2	65	33	13	13	Master's
Teacher 3	51	31	31	26	Master's
Teacher 4	37	16	3	3	CAGS
Teacher 5	45	22	11	11	Master's
Teacher 6	28	6	3	2	CAGS

Teacher 7	54	33	27	10	Master's
Teacher 8	43	21	13	15	Master's
Teacher 9	46	20	5	2	Master's
Teacher 10	38	15	5	10	Master's
Teacher 11	62	25	13	18	Master's
Teacher 12	30	8	3	3	Master's
Teacher 13	43	20	6	19	Master's

ABOUT THIS BOOK

All the exemplary educators expressed how hard it was to do their job well. In keeping with the notion of burnout as the "reduction of fuel . . . to nothing through use," the teachers also shared where they find the fuel needed to foster success.[13] In one way or another, each practitioner has been able to figure out how to meet the job's challenges. Given the wealth of strategies that have proven successful for these practitioners, I hope you gain a number of ideas to inform your own teaching practice, whether you are a preservice teacher, a professor in higher education, a K–12 educator, or you are an out-of-school-time professional.

The book is specifically designed to spur thinking and conversation about what supports and inhibits educator success. I would like to emphasize that the shared information represents the perceptions of the exemplary practitioners involved in the study. While the teacher comments do not presume to be the final word on exemplary educators, avoidance of burnout, or teaching excellence, they do provide an avenue to open fruitful dialogue about these important topics.

The book is organized into three sections, and some ideas overlap from one chapter to another. Part I explores how the exemplary teachers see their role as educators. Part II examines the key relationships that influence the exemplary practitioners' teaching experience. Part III identifies the ways the exemplary teachers' personal practices and skills contribute to their teaching outcomes. Appendixes with exercises, free resources, and additional information follow.

Feel free to read the book in whatever order makes the most sense to you. The book is deliberately designed for that purpose. You can use the material for your own professional development and/or as a group discussion with colleagues, as a faculty team (grade level or subject matter), or whole staff.

Educators are busy. Consequently, you'll find that each chapter contains short passages built around teacher quotes and exercises.

Teaching is personal, and you have your own way of doing things. Therefore, I offer lots of opportunity throughout each chapter for you to think about how the offered ideas either fit or do not fit with your own teaching practices. The prompts are designed to invite you to consider what you think and believe as an educator. I do this because, as you know, making a personal connection to the content makes learning easier, more meaningful, and memorable.

When reading, you will have a chance to hear what the exemplary educators have to say about what they do and why they do it. You will also be able to explore how, considered individually and together, the exemplary educators' beliefs, priorities, decisions, and actions help to foster their success. While not a quick fix, I hope that, by providing the exemplary educators' thoughts and feelings, you are afforded the opportunity to view your own educational practice through a variety of lenses. Through this process, you may gain greater insight into your work as an educator, what you tend to do, and your rationale for doing so.

The featured teachers provide insight into what is behind the curtain of their exemplary educator performance. In this time of high teacher attrition, we need to share ideas about how to succeed in the teaching profession. I hope you find it useful, supportive, and helpful to your work. I also hope this book inspires further research into educator well-being and teacher excellence and that it is a springboard for greater understanding of exemplary teacher practice while avoiding burnout.

I

How Teachers See Their Work

You may quickly notice when reading the teacher quotes in this book that the educators are acutely aware of the difficulties and challenges they experience when teaching. They agree with the research: "teaching is one of the most demanding and stressful professions."[1] That said, you will also likely see that the teachers are appreciative of the power and influence that comes with the position.

The following three chapters, "Teacher Power," "The Gift of Providing a Fresh Start," and "Meaning and Purpose," explore how the teachers' view of their role affects their energy, experience of burnout, and ability to cultivate success. This exploration begins with, of all things, considering the life of a turtle.

SEA TURTLES AND HUMANS

After emerging from their protective shells and successfully completing a mad dash to the sea, turtles figure out how to survive, live, and thrive on their own through instinct, trial, and error. In sharp contrast, humans are a social species, highly dependent on caregivers from birth, requiring positive connections with others in order to thrive throughout a lifetime. As Jordan explains, "our neurobiological wiring is relational. We grow and flourish in connection. We are interdependent beings."[2]

Our lives are lived through interaction within a relational and cultural world. We affect and are influenced by people around us. Lieberman describes the essential role of social connection, love, and belonging in the human experience: "Being socially connected is a need with a capital N. . . . Love and belonging might seem like a convenience we can live without, but our biology is built to thirst for connection because it is linked to our most basic survival needs."[3]

You can test this out for yourself by thinking about one of your biggest successes in life:

- Consider the strengths, skills, and attributes that you used in pursuit of that success. Who helped you identify and refine your talents?
- What did you have to overcome in order to achieve that level of success? What did you do? How did you do it? Who else was involved at different points in the process?
- What were some of the situational variables involving others that gave you an advantage? How did they help?

It is likely that your success cannot be completely extricated from relationships with others. Our lives exist within a web of complex relational ties. This fundamental relational context has the power to influence teaching experiences.

What follows are brief highlights from the groundbreaking findings of researchers Amy Wrzesniewski, Jane Dutton, Gelaye Debebe, and Adam Grant. They all study how people's perceptions of their work influences their experiences of their work. As you read on, consider how each may relate to you and your work as an educator.

HOW DO YOU DESCRIBE YOUR WORK?

Keep your answer to this question in mind while reading about Yale University's Amy Wrzesniewski, University of Michigan's Jane Dutton, and George Washington University's Gelaye Debebe's famous hospital study involving custodians who worked in the same hospital.[4] It is important to note that all the custodians interviewed had the exact same job description. Interestingly, during the research interviews, the custodians described their role in very different ways and, correspondingly, did their custodial job differently.

Wrzesniewski, Dutton, and Debebe found the "employees [constructed] their own experiences of the meaningfulness in their work by thinking about and performing their jobs in particular ways."[5] For example, when they asked the custodians about their role in the organization, some custodians responded with their technical job description for the custodial position. Those custodians went on to describe the job as not particularly satisfying and not requiring very high-level skills.[6]

Other custodians described their role in the organization quite differently. They responded with answers like "I'm an ambassador for the hospital. Or, in one case, I'm a healer."[7] Some custodians described the various ways their custodial work served as the foundation of the hospital's success. They shared, for example, how their cleaning efforts rid the hospital environment of harmful bacteria and other dangers that could inhibit the health of not only patients but also hospital staff. The custodians' thoughts, feelings, and beliefs about their work affected their experiences of their work, job satisfaction, enjoyment, level of engagement, and how the job of custodian was conducted.[8]

With Wrzesniewski, Dutton, and Debebe's findings in mind, you might ask yourself,

- How do I currently view my job as an educator?
- What do I tend to talk about when I describe my work to others?
- How might my current understanding of my work influence my experience of my work?
- What else might also be true about the work I do that, if more clearly articulated, could enhance my appreciation of the value and influence of my efforts?

WHY DOES YOUR WORK MATTER?

Research suggests what people see, think, feel, and believe about their work affects their experience of it.[9] These influences also affect whether the work produces or drains energy for people. University of Pennsylvania researcher Adam Grant found,

> Although many employees do work that has a meaningful impact on others, all too often, they lack a vivid understanding of how their efforts make a difference. My studies demonstrate that employees work harder, smarter, longer, more generously, and more productively when they can see how their work

affects others. . . . [Their] spikes in motivation are driven uniquely by an enriched appreciation of how one's work benefits others.[10]

What follows are three quotes that emerged during the exemplary teacher interviews. While reading them, consider how they relate to Grant's and Wrzesniewski, Dutton, and Debebe's research. In addition, examine how the quotes below might be similar to or different from what you think, feel, and believe about the work you do:

> Deborah highlighted the value and benefit of teaching a particular subject matter:
>
>> It's a gift . . . when you teach a child to read. You have given them an opportunity to be successful.
>
> Patty spoke about her ability to affect how students feel about going to school and her satisfaction with providing students with the foundational skill set they will need for future success:
>
>> I love feeling like the kids have had a good experience in that, when they think about their early years, they are going to say, "Kindergarten was great!" . . . I think . . . it's the idea that you're kind of nurturing that little person and helping them get a good start. It's *really, really* exciting for me.
>
> Kayla discussed the scope of influence that teachers have on their students:
>
>> Teaching gives me satisfaction [in that I] know that . . . I touch a life. So when I can say, . . . "I helped this kid who was having difficulty get what he needed," or . . . "Look at her. She is smiling, and she wasn't before," . . . It's not just about the academics. I . . . know that I touched somebody's life, and I know that hopefully each child is better off from having had me.

- How might Deborah, Patty, and Kayla's view of their work influence their experiences of their work?
- In order to make the following three chapters more meaningful, consider how different aspects of your work benefits others.

Chapter One

Teacher Power

In this chapter, the exemplary teachers explain how they understand and use the power inherent in the teaching role. This deep appreciation of their significant influence on others is a source of motivation and energy. It acts as fuel affecting the educator's capacity to negotiate the job's many challenges.

Suzy spoke about how hard it is to be a teacher:

> It is an incredibly challenging job, and it is becoming more challenging with every year, [with] the dynamics of children that are coming in with their *exceptionally* diverse needs, so [to be successful] you must love what you do; you must be passionate about helping children be the best that they can be. . . . It's oftentimes a thankless job, so you really have to . . . be driven from within to help others. And I think, first and foremost, that's where we start.

One way the exemplary teachers help their students is through the recognition and responsible use of teacher power. These teachers are highly aware of their ability to influence their students' lives inside and outside the classroom. In a variety of ways, all expressed deep understanding of their power to affect their students, moment by moment, throughout the day, during a week, over the course of the year, and in life beyond. The teachers recognize that their actions profoundly influence their students' lives in the short and long term. The educators take the power of their role very seriously. With awareness, they intentionally use it to help their students thrive.

- What are some things that immediately come to mind when you think about how you use your power to help your students?

What follows are examples of how the exemplary educators understand and embrace teacher power.

HANDLING MISBEHAVIOR

Kim spoke about the power of teacher-student interactions in whole-class settings. She knows students watch and learn from how she interacts with each student. She works hard to not be perceived as having favorites. Kim also handles misbehavior quietly, one on one. She understands that how she speaks to a student in front of others in the class influences that student's relationship with classmates. Kim said, if the teacher is

> verbally correcting [a] student in front of everybody else, I find [the student] becomes the scapegoat. . . . They are the student that other children are less likely to want to choose as a partner. . . . Noticing that earlier on in my career . . . [I] thought [a lot] about how I could help that [from happening]. . . . [I realized] I need to make [handling misbehavior] a private thing, between the student and I, so it . . . [doesn't negatively affect] how the other students treat that [student]. . . .
>
> I don't think [students] should ever [think], "Well, this is her favorite." . . . I think every child should go home thinking that they are my favorite.

Kim's belief is consistent with McGrath and Noble's findings that students observe and learn from watching the relationships their teacher has with different students; what they notice in teacher-student exchanges affects classroom student-student relationships.[1] A student's relationship with classmates has broad ramifications affecting life experience and performance in and out of school in the short and long term.

- Consider how your relationships with classmates affected your growth and development in the short and long term.
- What might be some consequences if students feel their teacher has favorites and least favorites?

Suzy used the word *mortifying* for how public reprimands from teachers can affect some students. She described how negative teacher-student experiences can have a long-lasting impact: "Those things stay with us, and . . . if the teacher has this much power, and we do, we have to appreciate that and respect that."

- How does your awareness of your power affect your decision-making and behavior in the classroom?

THE STUDENTS ARE WATCHING

The teacher is always modeling. During good days and bad, the students are watching.[2] June, Katie, and Jillian underscored this powerful feature of the teaching role.

June shared an experience from very early in her career that still influences her daily teaching practice. At the time, June had just switched from teaching elementary school to high school in a large nearby city. She described how she would have conversations with her students to get to know them better:

> I had a lot of girls [who] would talk [with me] about [their time] in Cambodia, the Khmer Rouge . . . telling me the horror stories. [One day] we were talking about what they wanted to do [after high school], and one girl said to me . . . "I want to be like you when I grow up." . . . I was like (a surprised facial expression).
>
> You know, [back then] I didn't realize I had that kind of influence. . . . I remember thinking to myself, "*Wow!*" . . . I never thought . . . that they [might] want to be like me. . . . I still, to this day remember that one because . . . it threw me. . . . I wasn't expecting that. . . . "I have . . . more of an impact than I thought" . . . [In that moment, I realized,] "Huh, they see more in us than we think that they see in us."

Part of June's self-awareness and self-management in teaching arises from this long-ago conversation and her appreciation of the power of teacher modeling. June went on to proudly say that the student "ended up going in the navy, . . . and she was the first female to be on the [ship]!"

- What do you think your students learn from who you are as a person?

Katie similarly appreciates the power of teacher modeling. This awareness informs her behavior throughout the day. For example, she is highly aware of her manner and tone when interacting with students and when speaking with colleagues:

> I think you are the role model for [students], whether you're teaching or you're talking to somebody in the hallway, so you should really pay attention to what

you're saying and how you are saying it because [the students] pick up on everything. . . . How [staff] treat each other [is important]. . . . We are a close [grade-level teaching] team so we [often] are laughing together, and [the students] see that, which I think is great! . . . I think we are a role model when we are [teaching and when we are] not teaching, too, *definitely*.

- How might seeing their teachers enjoying their work with one another affect students?
- What are some examples of how you and your colleagues model positive relationships for your students?

Jillian also spoke about how important it is for students to have positive role models in their lives. To that end, the fact that she loves learning and is continuing her education at night and on weekends is well known to her class:

I tell them a lot about myself. I am in school right now, and I tell them, "You know, I have homework every night." I tell them that I work really hard, and they see that, so they have that role model. . . . I'll tell [my students about] the other [grade-level] teacher, as well. She [also] went to [graduate] school [on weekends]. We [both] work really hard. . . . By showing them . . . role models, . . . they have somebody to look up to.

- What are some ways Jillian's students might be affected by hearing her talk about how much she loves learning and how hard she works on her homework for her advanced degree?
- In what ways do you think adult role models influence student development?

EXPLICIT TEACHER COMMUNICATION AND MESSAGING

The teachers use their power to explicitly set the tone for learning in their classroom. All the exemplary educators talk with their students about high expectations and hard work. This intentional teacher messaging may be another clue to their teaching success. In *Schools That Learn*, Senge and colleagues highlight how positive messaging, intentional teacher language, and clear communication supports high student achievement.[3]

Wanda shared how, on the first day of school, she explicitly explains to her fourth-grade students that she will not accept mediocrity. They have a conversation about the word *mediocrity* and she tells her students, "I don't teach you (gestures low) because I do not want to insult you. I want to teach up here (gestures high), and I want you to rise. I want you to find your own ladder. And, I want you to get there. And, I am going to help you every step of the way. But I *will not* accept work without effort. I *will not* accept a lack of quality. And I *will not* accept *you* accepting *that*."

- What do you tend to do and say during the first month of school to communicate your expectations and establish your classroom culture?
- What are some things Wanda's students might think and feel when they hear what she has to say about mediocrity on the first day of school?

The educators maintain their high expectations even when students come from difficult circumstances outside school. Katie acknowledged the challenges some of her students face when she said, "I don't know how they get out of bed in the morning. It's *that* sad." She expressed that she has a strong desire to support, help, and show kindness to her students, and maintaining high expectations for each of them is one way of doing that.

Knowing her students well helps Katie provide the level of academic challenge that supports each student's growth and development. Katie said, "When they're here, they're not thinking about home. They're happy . . . they're in a good place for the most part, and they have . . . a belief in themselves. . . . They are doing *great* things, and they're proud of themselves."

Maintaining high teacher expectations gives students an opportunity to focus their attention and experience the satisfaction of hard-won academic achievement that serves to influence the students' positive sense of themselves. Students are afforded the chance to strive, learn, and succeed while doing something difficult. Katie's relationships with and understanding of her students gives her the ability to encourage and support each student effectively when they are learning. Katie went on to say, "They have to still rise. *And they will.* They *know* that you have faith in them, and you believe in them, and *they will* rise to the occasion."

- What are some of the messages you intentionally and consistently communicate to your students throughout the year?

BURNOUT AND THE DESIRE TO HELP

All the exemplary teachers strive to recognize and understand the challenges their students face. The teachers also consistently expressed a grounded and focused desire to help their students. This compassionate orientation that emphasizes helping may provide insight into their ability to avoid burnout. An explanation of this comes from recent research in neuroscience.

Neuroscientist Tania Singer of the Max Planck Institute for Human Cognitive and Brain Sciences conducted research comparing compassion and empathy and found surprising results. Empathy and compassion "rely on different biological systems and brain networks."[4] Compassion's neural signature was qualitatively different than empathy. While compassion related to positivity, empathy related to pain.

Generally speaking, empathy relates to our ability to take another person's perspective and recognize that person's emotions. It involves attunement between people and often evokes emotion in response to seeing another person's distress. It is important to note, this empathic resonance does not happen in all situations. For example, it can be blocked when we believe someone has acted unfairly and also when we view someone as *not us* or *not in our tribe*.[5]

To better understand the experience of compassion, Emma Seppala, science director of Stanford University's Center for Compassion and Altruism Research and Education, invites consideration of the following example: "Imagine a day when things aren't going well for you—you spilled your coffee on yourself, and it's raining. And then a friend calls who's having a true emergency in their life, and you jump up and go help them immediately. What happens to your state of mind in that moment? All of a sudden you have high energy; you're completely at their service."[6]

Compassion differs from empathy in significant ways. Mahoney describes how "empathy is generally a more instinctive and reactive emotional state, whereas compassion extends beyond empathy to some sort of positive action or mindful intervention."[7] Singer distinguishes empathy and compassion by stating,

> When I empathize with the suffering of others, I feel the pain of others; I am suffering myself. This can become so intense that it produces empathic distress in me and in the long run could lead to burnout and withdrawal. In contrast, if we feel compassion for some[one] else's suffering, we do not necessarily feel

with their pain but we feel concern—a feeling of love and warmth—and we can develop a strong motivation to help the other.[8]

This emphasis on helping is evident in Rachel's comments about what contributes to successful educational outcomes: "I think you have to love teaching and love kids. And [you have to] *want* to help them in order to really be a successful teacher and for these kids to succeed."

- Consider some ways compassion and the "strong motivation to help" informs your teaching practice.
- Generally speaking, in what ways might the quality of teacher-student relationships influence teacher compassion and vice versa?

Chapter Two

The Gift of Providing a Fresh Start

Nearly all the educators spoke about the importance and power of providing students with a fresh start. Whether it is saying something like "Let's start the day over" after a student's particularly rough morning or whispering a gentle reminder at the end of a tough day that "Tomorrow is a new day," the educators explicitly convey an openness to student errors in judgment, mistake making, and the possibility of change. This chapter includes what they shared about the influential potential of starting anew.

- In your experience, what does the gift of a fresh start look like, sound like, and feel like?

Some of the exemplary teachers shared that they explicitly emphasize this opportunity with their students in the beginning of the year, thus opening the door to the students' reinvention of themselves. Suzy said,

> I truly believe this—when [students] walk in this room, [they've] got a clean slate. And I tell them that. I say, "I don't care what happened in [other grades]. We are starting fresh." . . . I want them to know that. And, I want them to own that. So the only way that they are going to know that and own that is if I truly believe it. . . .
>
> I believe that everyone deserves a fresh start. And sometimes, when [the students] know [it is possible], that's all they need.

- What might Suzy's students be thinking and feeling when they hear her invitation to start fresh at the beginning of the school year?

- Everyone has many different parts of who they are. How might Suzy's invitation influence the students' decision-making regarding who they want to be when they are in her classroom?
- What does that explicit message convey to the students about Suzy as a teacher and as a person?

As Suzy said, in order for this to work well, teachers must fully believe it themselves. The teacher must believe the students are more than their past mistakes. The teacher also must be open to student growth and transformation.

- What do you think about people's ability to change?

Wanda expressed how important it is to hold a flexible view of students and seek a deeper understanding of them. She shared the example of teaching a student with an extremely negative reputation:

> I saw goodness in him. I did see goodness. I saw sparks of goodness. It wasn't goodness all the time, but it was sparks. And I thought, "Where there is a spark, you can create a fire, just consistently helping him to find the right way."
>
> And when I looked into his background, . . . it was very sad. . . . He was on the street a lot. When you are a street kid, you have to develop these mechanisms to survive. He was only 9 years old, and he was out at night, you know. . . . He just missed out on a portion of his childhood because he went from being a little kid to being a street-smart punk. And I am *not* going to have that in my class.
>
> I want to find the little boy in him. I want to find the goodness in him. And how do you get that from someone? You respect them. I think you respect them. I think it really comes down to respect and empathy and praise.

- How might Wanda's approach of curiosity, respect, empathy, and praise have influenced her student's experience of school?
- Have you had a situation similar to Wanda's? If so, what helped you be successful?

Kim shared an example of a time when a fresh start served to shift a student's trajectory in school. The student's past teachers told Kim that he was a troublemaker. They told her how he had gotten caught "doing sneaky things" and "telling lies" in past years. Early in her school year with this student,

Kim began to notice some of the same behaviors described by colleagues. She immediately talked with the student about it and made his mother aware of it:

> Right away, that student picked up on [the fact that] . . . this is no nonsense. This isn't a place for me to fool around. . . . The next day, when the student came in, [I made sure] it was like nothing had happened. We'd been there. We've done that. It's a new day—we're going to start fresh. [We are going to] start over.
>
> The student was very intelligent, and I just continued to treat him as the intelligent student he was. [I kept] challenging him. . . . He realized that . . . I am not going to let him get away with that [other] stuff. . . . I actually told him, . . . "I know you are better than that. You are more capable than that. And I am not letting you get away with less." And he rose to the occasion. He had a wonderful year.

As highlighted in Chapter 1, the language teachers choose to use with students and the messages they send to students make an impact.[1] With that in mind, what might the student have thought and felt when Kim told him, "I know you are better than that. You are more capable than that. And I am not letting you get away with less"?

- Think of some examples when you provided a student with a fresh start. What happened? What helped?
- What are some of the consequences when a teacher does not give a student the gift of a fresh start? How can it affect the teacher? How can it affect the student? In what ways can it affect that student's relationship with classmates? What or who else can it influence?

PRECONCEIVED IDEAS ABOUT STUDENTS

This notion of a fresh start also relates to how the educators approach learning about their students. Most of the teachers shared that they intentionally do not read all provided prior teacher information before teaching their students. They do read any individualized education plan (IEP) requirements and other information of that ilk, but most expressed a strong need to form their own views of students without the input of previous educators. June said,

> I don't want preconceived notions of [students]. [The student] could have had a really bad year for whatever reason, whether it was a teacher-student conflict or something going on at home. . . . I don't want to have a preconceived notion of a student and already kind of have them red-flagged as being a pain in the neck . . . because then I would wait for [the] behavior or expect [certain] behavior. . . .
>
> I've learned not to seek [out information from prior teachers] ahead of time. Just start with a clean slate every year. (pause) And, for the kids, too, they want to start out fresh.

One teacher's negative experience with a student, widely shared with other staff, potentially causes other educators to be on the lookout for the negative behavior. Although perhaps intended as a kindness from one teacher to another, it has unintended negative consequences affecting educator expectations and perception that can affect student growth and development.

As soon as a human sees another human, each person makes conscious and subconscious split-second decisions about how to act and react. This decision-making process is informed in part by the context and what each person believes is true about the other. We rely on our beliefs and understandings to know what to do and how to treat others.[2] As June expressed, being told by a colleague to be on the lookout for something negative can foster a teacher's readiness to see previously described problems and student deficits instead of the student's existing strengths, skills, and potential.

Teachers cannot pay close attention to everything happening in the classroom, even if it is right in front of them. Humans are limited. You can try this out yourself. Right now, it is not possible for you to closely look at your hands while also reading this page while also seeing your environment clearly. Feel free to experiment with your focused attention: Intentionally move it from noticing what your hands look like to what the letters look like on the page to your environment and back again. This exercise demonstrates the narrow scope of our focused attention. Consider the way a teacher's naturally limited view affects different aspects of classroom life.

- How do you decide what to focus on when teaching?

Moment by moment, we each make conscious and subconscious decisions about where to place our attention. One way we each negotiate movement through our complex world is through expectations.[3] Humans naturally anticipate experience. For example, imagine if, at the end of a wet, cold, and wintery day of school, a colleague walked in and warned others about to depart, "Be careful out there. The parking lot is really icy. There are some super slippery spots. I almost wiped out three times!" It is likely people who heard that warning might soon be seen in the parking lot with their gaze toward the ground, looking carefully where they place their feet, altering their typical gait and walking speed. In anticipation of the possibility of slipping and falling, they use their focused attention to stay safe.

We each have established and powerful brain networks created over time that provide the rationale for what captures attention and holds our focus in a given situation. In schools, when teachers are warned to expect a forthcoming negative experience with a student, it cultivates a readiness to notice anything in the environment that triggers the anticipated experience.[4] June describes this when she said she might have a student "red-flagged as being a pain in the neck. . . . I would wait for [the] behavior or expect [certain] behavior."

- What do you think June meant when she said "red-flagged"? In what ways does it relate to expectations?

Another important variable is confirmation bias. Repeatedly, researchers find that people tend to seek information that confirms existing beliefs while ignoring or devaluing conflicting or contradictory information.[5] According to Eberhardt, "confirmation bias is a mechanism that allows inaccurate beliefs to spread and persist."[6] It also informs and influences what people notice, pay attention to, and remember.[7] Taken together, these natural human tendencies have powerful implications when considering how negative student and parent reputations develop and spread in schools.

- Has a colleague ever told you to "be on the lookout for ___"? If so, what are some things that helped you see beyond that colleague's negative view of the student or parent?

Rachel, an upper-grade-level teacher, spoke about how she works hard to remain open and not create preconceived ideas about students based on reputations, *even if* she has heard teachers sharing negative things about her students since kindergarten. She emphasized valuing and remembering that children grow, mature, and change over time. Students can even change a great deal over the course of one short summer break.

- How might this commitment to providing a *clean slate* affect an educator's experience of teaching? How could it influence educational outcomes?

THE TEACHER'S CLASSROOM CULTURE

The educators' comments conveyed a recognition and appreciation of how teacher-student power dynamics and different teachers' relational responses influence what aspect of each student is amplified.[8] For example, June said, "We know that [students] respond differently to different teachers." Behavior arises within a relational and a cultural context. In many ways, the participants referenced how important it is to be curious about who students can become in a different classroom environment and with a different teacher.

Each teacher-student relationship arises within a classroom environment. Each classroom's cultural environment or the "way we do things around here" is largely established and maintained by the teacher.[9] This personal process is informed in part by the teacher's beliefs, biases, likes, and dislikes arising from the educator's cultural background (e.g., socioeconomic status, ethnicity, schooling, personality, age, gender, social class, etc.).[10]

Gay suggests a person's culture is an anchor for all expressive behaviors (thinking, relating, speaking, writing, performing, producing, learning, and teaching).[11] It can be helpful to remember that the cultural backgrounds of teacher and students are in play throughout all schooling processes. It affects what each person sees, says, thinks, feels, and does. To explore this topic further, please see appendix D and the information listed under Bias, Implicit Cognition and Educational Equity in appendix F.

- In what ways is your cultural background similar to your students'? How does it differ? How do the similarities and differences influence how you see and understand each of your students?
- What's your hunch about how your similarities and differences may influence how each of your students see and experience you?

Gay emphasizes the importance of understanding the detailed workings of cultural influence in order to create equitable schools where all students thrive.[12] Teacher decisions, such as furniture configuration, lesson organization, behavioral expectations, classroom management, and class discourse, are informed by what feels right and comfortable to the teacher.[13]

The teacher's classroom culture may be more familiar to and comfortable for some students than others. Katie shared an example of this:

> I have . . . a student who had a *really* hard time [at school] last year, and this year he is doing awesome! . . . I think it's [because] it's more structured [in my classroom]. . . . I think he needed the structure, and his teacher last year was a wonderful person, . . . but she's all over the place, and he couldn't handle that, so he had a *really* hard time last year because . . . just because . . . that's her personality and she's just got so much going on. . . . It's the way it is [in her classroom. And that was hard for him]. But in here, he's been excellent. . . . He had a couple little issues but *nothing* like last year.

- Generally speaking, what are some ways a classroom's culture affects student behavior?
- Have you ever had a student behave differently in your class than in another setting? What are some variables that may have affected that behavioral shift?

The classroom's cultural environment, along with all relationships within the class community, has a profound influence on each person's behavioral decision-making. Deborah highlighted the importance of remembering and recognizing this powerful influence when she spoke about wanting to be open to who students can become in her classroom environment. Deborah and other teachers also spoke about the need to sometimes change aspects of the classroom environment to better address students' needs throughout the year:

> I try to make my own judgments and decisions [about] kids based upon my classroom routines and my teaching style and how kids adapt to that or adhere to that or how I have to adapt to adhere to them. So I try not to put too much weight in what others will say to me [about a student's past behavior in their classrooms]. . . . I make my own opinions based on how [the students] come in and just go from there.

- Think of when you have adapted routines or your teaching style to help support students' success in your classroom?

UNDERMINING NEGATIVE STUDENT REPUTATIONS

- Think of some students who have had pervasive negative reputations. How might negative reputations have shaped those students' growth and development over time?
- Have you ever been in a situation or environment when you believed that people thought poorly of you? If so, in what ways did it influence your behavior?

Wanda described that, when a student has a poor reputation, it sometimes acts like an "invisible sign" that educators see hanging around a student's neck that says, "I'm naughty," or, "I'm bad." A student's negative reputation informs the student's relationships with the adults in the school. A pervasive negative reputation also affects who that student can become in the school setting. Wanda works hard to provide her students with a fresh start, not only in her classroom, but in her school, as well.

Sometimes Wanda uses the identification and celebration of student successes as a vehicle to shift the prevailing reputations about some of her students. Wanda shared an example of a time when she sent her fourth-grade student, who had a long-standing pervasive negative reputation, with his excellent academic work in hand, "down to his last year's teacher, and I would [also] send him to the principal." Wanda described how her student looked when he returned to her classroom. He had a visible change. She said, "He would come back, and . . . the muscles were relaxed in his face. He wasn't tense."

These quick visits to past teachers and the school principal, where the student shares the successful project or test, provides the student with an opportunity to have multiple celebrations of his effort and growth. These interpersonal exchanges help amplify the student's awareness of and pride in his academic accomplishment. It gives the student a positive experience with these influential adults with whom he has had many negative interactions.

Importantly, each adult gains a positively augmented view of the student. Wanda's intentional process expands the breadth of information that the adults consider when they see this student—whom they previously labeled difficult and challenging—walking down the hall. It can provide a rationale to shift a habitual negative response to him to an authentically positive one.

- What difference might it make to Wanda's student if more adults greeted him with authentic positivity when they saw him walking down the hall?

How might it influence her student's response to adults? How might it affect her student's experience of school?
- What comes to mind when you consider the extent to which students receive a fresh start in your school setting? What is helpful to that aim? What could be done differently?

Chapter Three

Meaning and Purpose

During the research interviews, it became clear that the exemplary teachers' rationale for entering the field differed. Some reasons were seeing a family member's joy in being an educator, being taught by extraordinary and impactful positive teachers during childhood, wanting to be the opposite of the negative teacher(s) they experienced growing up, seeking a work life that involved children, wanting a job that required creativity and independence, being inspired by their faith to be of service to others, and/or deep knowing from an early age that they were born to be a teacher.

They also had different life experiences that led them to where they are now. Some went straight from college to teaching, and others had different careers (inside and outside education) before becoming a teacher. Although they have different reasons for becoming teachers and different life experiences that inform their teaching practices, they all find deep meaning and purpose in their work.

Importantly, when people actively find meaning and purpose in their work, it influences their experience of the work they are doing and the quality of the work done. It can also affect energy and well-being.[1] This chapter explores what the exemplary teachers had to say about the meaning and purpose they find in the teaching role. It concludes with conflicts some teachers faced when their deeply held values did not align with their school's practices.

- One way to explore meaning and purpose is to examine why you are doing what you are doing. With that in mind, what are some reasons you became an educator?
- What are some of the key influences that affected your journey to becoming an educator?
- What keeps you in education?

PAYING IT FORWARD

The meaning and purpose Debbie finds in her role comes from her own experiences as a student. Debbie had an extremely difficult home life as a child. She has a powerful lived experience of how a school's positive environment can transform a person's life trajectory. Debbie shared that, when she was growing up,

> school was where things were consistent and safe. . . . I buried myself there . . . Kids need that. . . . Kids need a place where things are consistent and safe and everything is okay. And that is what I think . . . drives me to have the relationships that I make with the kids. . . . I really appreciated the opportunity to have that as a kid, and so I need to pay it forward and *give that* as a teacher.

Debbie holds a deep appreciation for the teachers she had growing up. Those relationships continue to significantly influence Debbie's sense of herself as an educator. They also inform her compassionate response to the students in her care.

- In what ways does your educational experience growing up affect your teaching practice?
- How might your past relationships with teachers influence the meaning and purpose you find in your teaching practice?

STUDENTS' VISION OF WHAT LIFE CAN BE

One aspect of meaning and purpose that Kayla shared was how she could alter her students' vision of what their lives could be. She described the inequities in her students' experiences. Her students and their families do not begin or live with the same resources or have the same advantages. It is clear that, given unequal starting circumstances and embedded societal structures, the future is more open for some students than others. It is not a level playing field.

Kayla strives to nurture in her students a strong belief that they can be successful in life. She said,

> I have kids that just arrived here this year. They don't speak very much English. . . . I want little kids who may not know where their next meal is coming from [as well as] . . . the kids whose parents are doctors and lawyers. . . . I want to them to know hard work—trying. . . . You have to have [perseverance]. . . . [Years ago] I started using the word *college* [with] my first-grade students. . . . I want them to [think about their future].

Kayla cultivates a sense of belonging for all her students by putting a high value on kindness and working together as a team. She said, "I *really* want the class to help each other to progress—no 'ha-ha, you didn't get that' [when a student makes a mistake]. . . . I also want them to [have and experience] a positive attitude towards being in school and . . . towards each other."

Kayla knows teaching offers her a chance to affect her students' beliefs about their ability to be successful in her classroom and in the future. Kayla wants to create a safe learning environment, and she works hard to nurture each student's skill development. Her relationships with her students support those aims.

Kayla self-identifies as a White woman. She shared that her grandparents emigrated from Ireland and Poland. Growing up, Kayla heard stories about the struggles and injustices her four grandparents experienced in the United States.

- In what ways do you think Kayla's background influences her teaching practice and priorities? How does your cultural background influence your teaching practice and priorities?
- What else could Kayla say and do to support educational equity and social justice?
- How can a student's experience of belonging influence student behavioral decision making in and out of learning situations? What are some ways your sense of belonging has influenced your behavior with others?

To further explore this topic, please see the related links listed under Bias, Implicit Cognition, and Educational Equity in Appendix F.

LIFE SKILLS AND STUDENTS' SELF-CONCEPT

Having students learn the required subject matter is clearly a high priority for the exemplary teachers. Fostering student content mastery is one way the educators find meaning and purpose in their work. At the same time, the teachers also clearly understand their ability to shape who each student becomes as a person. The teachers shared thoughts about the power they have to affect their students' life skills and self-concepts. These provide another dimension of meaning and purpose to their work as educators.

- In addition to teaching subject matter, what other aspects of the role provide you with meaning and purpose?

One way Katie finds meaning and purpose in her work lies in her ability to nurture and develop each student's life skills in general and kindness in particular. Katie shared that her students need to know

> how to treat other people. We . . . work a lot in cooperative groups and in teams. [The students might] not like everybody, but [they] need to get along. I really want them to learn . . . what . . . they used to call citizenship. Citizenship [is] being kind to other people, getting along with other people. Of course I want them to be good in math and reading and writing, . . . but I think being a good person is huge. . . . You have to [learn that] . . . no matter where you go and what you do in life, you're going to have to know how to get along with other people.

- What are some ways you help students learn how to get along with others?

Jillian also places a high value on interpersonal understanding and relationship skill building. To support their development, Jillian has her students work together (pairs, trios, and small groups) at least once on every academic task. She intentionally holds high expectations for all, "even those [students] you have heard those [negative] things about." Jillian's students practice and hone interpersonal skills through their academic work with others. They also learn about themselves during those interactions.

Jillian's comments reflect her understanding of how relationships influence learning and change. She appreciates how her structure of classroom tasks affects how each student grows and develops during their time with her. It is important to Jillian to positively influence what her students believe about who they are and what they can do. To Jillian, every student "should leave your classroom stronger and more confident than they entered."

- What are some ways you support your students' sense of themselves as people as well as learners?
- In what ways do you think classroom relationships provide students with information affecting their self-concepts?

Kim also finds meaning and purpose in being able to influence her students' foundational sense of themselves. She understands that relationships affect inner confidence. Consequently, Kim works hard to provide a trusting relational context; she strives to nurture an openness and willingness to take learning risks in each student. Kim explained, "I found that [there seems] to be just this general, like underlying layer [that will] help all students be successful. If they had the [inner] confidence, they'd be willing to take more risks. And then, once [they're] taking those risks and finding successes, they are willing to keep working. And [part of it is] that they are trusting me more."

- Kim mixes the concepts of risk taking, trust, confidence, and relationships. How do you think these affect each other?
- What affects your inner confidence in different situations with different groups of people?

To Suzy, teaching students to use goals to support a life of meaning and purpose grounds her teaching practice. Teaching students about the importance of living a fully engaged life is a significant source of fuel for Suzy:

> I really want to instill in my students a passion for them to constantly be working towards a goal—long-term goals, short-term goals—make every day count. Make every day have meaning and purpose. We start our day off, every single day with [four things]: We sing, we dance, we exercise, and then we reflect—what do I want to accomplish today, what do I want to accomplish this week and this year. They just take a few minutes and think about it. . . .
>
> I think . . . we need to have goals in life. We need to be constantly working towards goals. Although they are young, I think now is the time to set that foundation. Don't just slide through life. Make every day have purpose.
>
> And then, you need to leave here exhausted. I tell them at the end of the day, "You should leave here exhausted. I go home exhausted, and that's because I have given it my all." And so whatever you do—if it's a . . . worksheet,

if it's a letter to a [senator], if it is a science fair project—*make it your best*. If you are putting your name on that, you need to be proud of it. . . . Putting [your] stamp on it (taps table). This is who I am. This is the best I am. I think those . . . are . . . important things.

- What do you most want your students to take away from their time spent with you?

The exemplary teachers appreciate that the position of educator brings with it an incredible opportunity to share subject matter that possibly sparks students' interest and profoundly shapes their trajectories. The educators also know they can affect a child's future by helping students believe in themselves, by creating an environment where students put forth full effort and see positive results, and by teaching learning habits that support a lifetime of high achievement.

The educators deeply value that they can play a helpful role in each student's life story. They know that their hard work matters and positively influences others. This awareness acts as an important source of energy and motivation. They clearly recognize the possibilities and power associated with their role. They have, as Grant puts it, a "vivid understanding of how their efforts make a difference."[2] This influences their approach to and experience of their hard work.

- What meaning and purpose do you find in your work?

CONFLICTING VALUES AND TEACHER DEMORALIZATION

As mentioned, all the exemplary teachers find deep meaning in their work, and they understand how their efforts positively influence others. This awareness fuels their energizing sense of purpose. While this appreciation of the inherent power of the role is helpful to their well-being, it can also fuel dissonance when their professional values differ from the job's requirements. According to Santoro's research, conflicting values can, over time, cause teacher demoralization[3]:

> The diagnosis of [teacher] demoralization characterizes the problem as a value conflict experienced as a result of policies, mandates, and school practices. The individual teacher has not failed. In demoralization, experienced educators

understand that they are facing a conflict between their vision of good work and their teaching context.[4]

Santoro suggests the school's administration can exacerbate the situation and "repel some of the strongest and most dedicated experienced teachers in their buildings, districts, and states" when the administrators respond "as if teacher dissatisfaction is the individual's problem."[5] Demoralization is not an individual teacher's problem relating to a depletion of their enthusiasm or energy. Instead, demoralization relates to a "fundamental change in the rewards available through the practice" of teaching.[6] While the same emotions (e.g., discouragement and depression) may accompany both burnout and demoralization, the latter is "better understood as a process of continually being frustrated in one's pursuit of good teaching."[7]

Kayla, June, and Deborah's professional values can be heard in the following comments. To begin, Kayla spoke of the dissatisfaction and hardship she experienced when her school adopted curricula that did not fit with the developmental needs of her students:

> When we switched our math program, we were told we *had* to do the math program. . . . I had a disconnect with my love of math when I was told I *had to* do something I didn't believe in. . . . When I was stuck [with that] program, I had two *very* difficult years. The hard part was . . . I was doing a program that wasn't developmentally right for my [students]. Each concept was taking longer to teach than it should have if I'd been able to do it, sort of, more my way. . . .
>
> When they would come to model [math lessons] for us, the gentleman who was modeling the lessons for this [math] program . . . couldn't get the [students] to do what [he] wanted. They just weren't ready yet. . . . It was very difficult.
>
> [With that math program], I felt I was reteaching and re-teaching and . . . re-teaching things. I finally had to say, "Okay, I can teach this [required] whole-class lesson, but in small groups, I am now going to do what I want." I actually implemented Friday . . . math centers. I said, "You know, . . . we are going to teach things my way [during centers]. I'll do the [required] program four days and then I will teach the concepts my way [on Fridays]." I had to make that change. . . . The kids needed it. . . .
>
> We also went from [a] balanced literacy [approach] to a basal reader program. Being told to do this [basal] program [was hard]. . . . [The] program [did] not meet all the needs of [all my students]. So I had a real disconnect when we did [the basal program] two years in a row. [They said], "Well, they

have leveled readers, [and] they have small group." And I said, "But your low level doesn't fit the needs of my kids."

- Have you ever been told to teach a program that did not fit your students' educational needs? If so, what was that experience like for you? What helped support your ability to negotiate that challenge?

For June, the school culture and overall teaching environment in a previous school district became so unhealthy she had to leave:

> It got to the point where Monday mornings I wanted to cry. . . . I hated my job. [So] I switched. I gave up all my seniority. I gave up everything. . . . I changed things. . . . And I tell people that, if you don't like where you are, figure it out—don't get stuck there. There's no need to go to work every Monday . . . dreading it. . . . I knew that it wasn't that I hated teaching; it was the environment. . . .
>
> [At that school, they had] one teacher . . . on the pedestal, so everyone else kind of felt lousy. . . . It was so dysfunctional there. . . . You have to be careful of that. . . . There was a model teacher for each grade level and everyone else was nothing. . . . But . . . everyone else [had something to offer]—this person had great classroom management, this person . . . was there every day, stayed [late, and was] . . . never absent, so everyone brings something to the plate! . . . I think a lot of times principals, . . . instead of looking at all the positive, try to find what's wrong, and [they] really pounce on those people. It was pretty wild [there]. And it still is, I guess. I just couldn't do it anymore.

- What are some ways that the school's environment influences your sense of well-being and ability to bring your best to your work?

Deborah described a town education policy decision that profoundly influenced how she could teach:

> I had 27 kids two years ago. I was by myself, with 27 [in first grade]. . . . They come from a kindergarten where they max out at 18 and they have two adults: a teacher and an aide. So here we are *screaming* from the rooftops, "How come kindergarten maxes out at 18 with two adults, but yet we have 27 children in our first grade, and we are alone, except for a half-hour a day where we have push-in reading support! . . . How come you can't open another first grade?" If you take seven from me and seven from her, and five from the other school, you've got a classroom. . . .
>
> But you can't do anything about that. . . . [Lining up,] the joke was, "Oh my god, your [student] line is never ending! . . . Look at your [student] line

compared to everybody else's [on the playground]. The first-grade lines are all the way to the [wall]!" It was like, "Yup."...

You put the names on all the mailboxes, and you don't have [enough] space. So, you add a few more up at the top.... You know it's not a choice. I can't shake some of these kids—they're mine.... It's going to be a long year, and we are going to make it work. I had to lose this [table] because I had to have another group of desks.... [Space was a real problem]—there wasn't much room to navigate around the room. But it wasn't [the students'] fault.... The higher-ups can't see what a problem that [policy is] going to create as far as what [the students] can learn.... There is only so much you can do with high numbers like that [in a room like this, with one teacher]. You can't reach everybody.

I lost sleep that year.... That was (pause) that was hard for me.... I don't like to feel like I can't get to everybody who needs it. That's the negative [of being a teacher]—you take that home with you. And if you don't take it home with you, and it doesn't matter to you, then, I don't really know if you belong here anymore because you're impacting a life [when you are a teacher]....

So then, you *have* to find the positive in it. And, you have to make it work. You find a way to do that.... [One thing I did was have] a parent reader who came in every morning just to listen to kids read.... That's what you [have to] do.... Try [to] find a way to make it positive because you can't change that negative [policy decision].

- Have you ever experienced a school policy decision that negatively influenced your work, but you had no ability to change it? How were you able to handle that situation? What did you find helpful?

In *Demoralized: Why Teachers Leave the Profession They Love and How They Can Stay*, Santoro provides a variety of steps teachers can take to mitigate demoralization.[8] Also, in order to prevent and reverse demoralization, Santoro suggests school administrators "be cognizant of and recognize the moral commitments teachers bring to their work. It means working with teachers to articulate the features of good work and to support ways that good work can be done in their classroom, school, district, and state."[9]

- How would you describe good work in education? What supports your ability to do good work? What gets in the way?
- Do you ever feel demoralized? If so, what are some factors that influence that experience? What helps?
- Do you ever feel burned out? If so, what are some factors that influence that experience? What helps?

II

The Central Role of Relationships

Teaching involves subject matter (*the what*), applied teaching techniques (*the how*), and people (*the who*). The focus of the next seven chapters is people. You will hear why the exemplary educators invest time and energy in relationship building as well as how they nurture relationships and negotiate relational challenges.

This part of the book includes Chapter 4, "Knowing Students Well"; Chapter 5, "Cultivating Positive Relationships With Students"; Chapter 6, "Negotiating Difficult Relationships With Students"; Chapter 7, "Investing in a Positive Learning Environment"; Chapter 8, "Connecting With Parents and Caregivers"; Chapter 9, "Relationships With Colleagues"; and Chapter 10, "The Administration of Schools." The foundation for this exploration of relationships begins with an invitation to participate in a thought experiment called "Two Scenarios About Crossing a Room."

SCENARIO 1 INSTRUCTIONS

Imagine the following scenario as fully as you can, so you can experience not only a greater depth of thoughts and feelings but also notice a physiological response:

> Imagine you are standing in a doorway. You begin walking into a relatively large room. The room is a comfortable temperature. It contains a few desks

and chairs. You notice that there is one person standing in a sunny spot by a far window. This person is looking out the window at the view.

The person is someone you know, with whom you have a somewhat negative relationship. The person is not dangerous but is someone you do not fully trust. You are not certain that it is safe to take risks with or show weakness to this person. You do not enjoy spending time with this person.

Do you have the person in mind?

Now, imagine that the person slowly gazes away from the window and toward you. The person notices you. You walk toward and greet this person.

Think carefully about your answers to the following prompts:

- What might you be thinking and feeling as you move toward this person?
- What might you look like while you walk?
- How might you greet this person? What might you say?
- How would you characterize your tone of voice?
- If people were watching you during this experience, how might they describe you?

Next, consider the following:

Someone else walks into the room and gives you both a tricky task that involves a skill set you have not fully developed and requires you to work together. How would you feel? What might you think? How might you respond? How do you imagine your work together might unfold?

SCENARIO 2 INSTRUCTIONS

As before, imagine the following scenario as fully as you can so you can experience not only a greater depth of thoughts and feelings but also a physiological response:

Like last time, you are standing in a doorway. You begin walking into a relatively large room with a comfortable temperature. It contains a few desks and chairs. There is one person standing in a sunny spot by a far window. This person is looking out the window at the view. It is a different person.

This time, the person is someone who you know, who you have a positive relationship with, who you trust, who you feel it is safe to take risks with and show weakness to. You enjoy spending time with this person.

Do you have the person in mind?

Now imagine that the person slowly gazes away from the window and toward you. The person notices you. You walk toward and greet this person.

Think carefully about your answers to the following prompts:

- What might you be thinking and feeling as you move toward this person?
- What might you look like while you walk?
- How might you greet this person? What might you say?
- How would you characterize your tone of voice?
- If people were watching you during this experience, how might they describe you?

Next, consider the following:

> Someone else walks into the room and gives you both a tricky task that involves a skill set you have not fully developed and requires you to work together. How would you feel? What might you think? How might you respond? How do you imagine your work together might unfold?

• When you compare the thought experiments, what are some things you notice about yourself in Scenarios 1 and 2?

Educators who have completed this exercise tend to share very different experiences in Scenarios 1 and 2. They describe how the nature of the two relationships amplified different aspects of who they are. The relational context affected how they looked, spoke, and moved, as well as their levels of connection, engagement, and interest when completing the work they were asked to do together. The relational context would influence what would get done during the tricky task and how the work was completed.

• These scenarios are rich with information. What are some things that you can take away from the exercises?

To link your experience with "Two Scenarios About Crossing a Room" to the information in chapters 4–10, notice what comes to mind when you consider your answers to the following questions:

• What connections can you make between your thought experiment experiences and

- teacher–student relationships
- teacher–parent or –caregiver relationships

- colleague–colleague relationships?
  - teacher–administrator relationships?
  - student–student relationships?

- What do you use to determine how to treat others?
- What do you use to determine how to treat people you don't know?
- How much like you do people need to be for you to want to get to know them?

Chapter Four

Knowing Students Well

All the exemplary educators cited their knowledge of students as a primary influence on their success as teachers. They expressed strong relational interest and interpersonal curiosity. In this chapter, the exemplary teachers explain why they want to know their students well and how that understanding influences their students' educational outcomes.

- In your experience, how does knowing students well influence your ability to reach and teach each of your students effectively?

An educator's level of interpersonal curiosity may relate to foundational beliefs about the teaching role. A person who has lower relational interest may view the teacher's role as more of a content-delivery person, educational technician, organizer of educational experiences and processes, or knowledge disseminator. In these instances, the relationship between teacher and student is not the highest priority.

- How does knowing students well fit within your educational priorities?

Barb spoke about how her knowledge of her students affects what and how she teaches each year. She provided a contrasting example to illustrate her approach. Many years ago, in late August, before the school year began, she overheard a teacher say that she had all her copies made for the entire year. This was before the teacher had met her students. To Barb, completing all copying for the entire year would not be useful because she feels she first needs to know her students. She also finds it helpful to hold an expectation that teaching methods and approaches will likely change over the course of the year to meet each student's needs:

> My goal is to figure out how I can get to know [each student] better. . . . What is going to work for [one student] . . . may not work for the next person. . . . I think [you need to be] open to saying to yourself, "What works for A, is not going to work for B, and I'm okay with that. . . . Now I've got to figure out what I need to do, so I can get that particular [student] to do what I need him to do or [how] to support [the student] in a different way." . . .
>
> I think [you need] to be [tuned into] who you have in front of you . . . That's the key. You need to know who's in front of you to be able to develop what you need to do in your classroom.
>
> Each classroom is so unique, [so the same things don't always work]. . . . I'm changing things all the time. And, I think [that's what] makes a good teacher: . . . [It's seeing] who you have before you set what you need to set up for that year or that week or for that month, per se, *and* it changes.

- In what ways might the expectation and readiness for change influence what Barb thinks and feels when teaching?
- Think of times when knowing your students supported your ability to make effective adaptations (small, medium, or large) that enhanced their educational outcomes.

Barb's comments about teaching align with Capp's description of the universal design for learning (UDL) approach. UDL is not a "one-size-fits-all curriculum" approach; instead, the educator thinks first about students' learning needs and then considers curriculum. Capp explains,

> The philosophy of UDL is based on the idea that there are multiple ways of representing knowledge (principle one), multiple ways students can demonstrate their understanding (principle two), and multiple ways of engaging students (principle three). . . . [UDL] principles are underpinned by nine guidelines and 33 checkpoints."[1]

With UDL, academic supports and scaffolds for all learners are integrated into each lesson plan from the beginning. UDL involves proactively planning for the success of all students.

- What are some helpful strategies you use when planning lessons for your students?

21ST-CENTURY SCHOOLING

All educators in the study spoke about how hard it is to do their job well. The complex challenge of meeting a broad range of student academic needs is a hallmark of 21st-century schooling in the United States.[2] The task asked of teachers is extremely difficult to accomplish. Knowing students well supports a teacher's ability to effectively address academic differences between students.

Suzy shared that, in her third-grade classroom, she has students reading on a kindergarten level all the way up to a fifth-grade level:

> [That] is the greatest challenge of teaching. . . . It's my job to make the day count for [each of my students.] . . . How do I make sure . . . my kindergarten reader feels just as good about her accomplishments and her successes as [another student] feels about, you know, finishing Harry Potter?
>
> I tell them all, . . . "We are all working at our own level, and we all have our own goals." It comes back to those goals. "What was the goal you made for today, for this week, for this school year—a long-range goal?" . . . We revisit those goals all the time. . . .
>
> I take [a student] aside, and I say, "Honey what was your goal for today? What was your goal for this week?" . . . [or] "What do you want to do this week?" . . . [Then I ask,] "Okay, what can I do to help you reach this goal?" . . . And then, (pause) just celebrate every little victory. . . . Yeah, little successes. . . . It is hard. There needs to be 10 [teachers] in here to really make it count. It's *hard*.

Suzy's knowledge of her students influences how student learning goals are created, pursued, and met in her diverse academic setting. It also provides the basis for her expectations for each student. Suzy described how important it was to have high expectations, saying, "It's everything. *Everything*. If you don't have high expectations for your students, why would they?"

- What do you use as the basis of your expectations for each student?

Kim also referenced the power of teacher expectations: "If you set the bar low, that's all they're going to reach; that's all they are going to achieve. They are not going to strive to do better, if they . . . think that you [think] 'Okay, great, you did all you can, and that's the end of it.'"

- Think of some examples that illustrate how your knowledge and understanding of students supported your ability to provide them with the appropriate challenge.
- If you do not know a student well, what do you use to determine your course of action with that student?

Pope, Reynolds, and Mueller suggest authentic relationship building as one way to interrupt the unhelpful and often unconscious generalizations and stereotypes that blur a complex understanding of each person.[3] Stanford University's Jennifer Eberhardt states, "[B]ias, even when we are not conscious of it, has consequences that we need to understand and mitigate. The stereotypic associations we carry in our heads can affect what we perceive, how we think, and the actions we take."[4]

UNDERSTANDING STUDENTS' BACKGROUNDS

While knowing students academically is important, Katie also highlighted the value of knowing and understanding the students' world in order to teach them well:

> You have to know the kids' backgrounds. They come from very different households. You have to know what's going on in their family unit—good, bad, indifferent. Who do they live with? How many siblings do they have? I mean, I have kids in here whose baggage is unbelievable. So, you have to know the baggage to know how to deal with the student. . . . If you don't care enough to find out, then you [can] make a pretty grave mistake when you're talking to a [student.] . . . So, to know them . . . is everything.

- Think of a time when you gained insight into behavior after learning more about the student's background. In what ways did your teaching practice shift with that additional information?

Barb's desire to really understand her students' background is influenced by her close relationship with her grandparents. She thinks about them often when teaching:

> My grandparents . . . came to this country and did not speak English. [They] worked really, really hard, . . . [so] I think I know where some of these kids [are coming] from. . . . I know what . . . my grandparents didn't have [and] the stories that they shared [about] how hard it was to write, how hard it was to

have a conversation with someone. . . . [Hearing about] those kinds of experiences have helped me be a better educator.

- How might that past relationship with her grandparents help Barb be a better educator?
- In what ways can cultural background similarities affect teacher-student relationship building?
- In what ways can cultural background differences affect teacher-student relationship building?

When educators understand their students' cultural backgrounds, it enhances the sophistication and accuracy of teacher interpretations of student behavior. Phillips and Carr suggest teachers go through a structured cultural-awareness process to enhance cultural proficiency and self-awareness. This experience can more clearly make known the typical aspects of a given culture. These norms often are unnoticed and unexamined if a person is a member of the dominant culture. Overall, it can lead to a more comprehensive and nuanced understanding of what occurs in the classroom.[5]

For example, culture has a strong influence on verbal and written communication. In some cultures, details precede answers to enhance clarity; in others, streamlined logical facts are favored to bolster clarity. If educators are culturally oriented to prefer the more succinct discourse style, then they may perceive negatively the more detailed answers and the students who employ them.[6]

- What are some of your preferences? In what ways do your preferences influence what happens in your classroom?

Katherine shared a lesson she learned early in her career about the value of understanding her students' cultural backgrounds. It still influences her teaching approach today. Katherine's example involved a student who was from another country "where it is disrespectful to look a teacher in the eye. But here, we want [students] to look at us when we are speaking to them because it is disrespectful when you don't look at someone."

In her description, Katherine highlighted how the student was attempting to show her the highest level of respect by averting his direct gaze. Katherine spoke about how important it was to learn this lesson of teacher interpretations of student behavior. She recognized that a mistaken interpretation of the motives behind the student's behavior could have broad ramifications.

- If Katherine had thought that the student was disrespectful, in what ways might that determination have influenced the nature and quality of their teacher-student relationship?
- How might it have affected that student's experience of school?
- What else might it have influenced?

Gaitan advocates for more mindful teacher discernment and cultural self-awareness as well as fewer quick categorizations and judgments, so fewer mistakes are made while teaching.[7] Cultural mismatches can lead to a multitude of misunderstandings of student responses, facial expressions, and behavior unless educators are well versed in their own and their students' cultural backgrounds.[8]

Teacher understanding of students' cultural backgrounds can also be used to accelerate student learning. In *Culturally Responsive Teaching and the Brain*, Zaretta Hammond explains how to leverage the cultural basis of students' ways of thinking and learning. Positive teacher acknowledgment and the thoughtful use of cultural information acts "as a scaffold [connecting] what the student knows to new concepts and content."[9] When teachers actively build on students' ways of knowing, they facilitate rigorous learning. Knowing students well and a positive class dynamic supports this process. For more about Hammond's culturally responsive teaching approach, please see the related links listed under Bias, Implicit Cognition, and Educational Equity in appendix F.

TEACHING IS A MESSY PROCESS

According to Brookfield, much of teaching and learning involves a great degree of uncertainty, even for the best educators; teaching is a messy process.[10] Knowing students well provides teachers with a greater breadth and depth of information that they can use for their complex educational decision-making. It influences the accuracy of teacher interpretations of student behavior in and out of structured learning situations and enhances the success of teacher interventions.

Rachel described how the knowledge of her students and nurturing positive relationships over time support her negotiation of the messiness of learning: "I think that whole thing of starting early to really get to know your kids is so important because there's so many different parts to the puzzle that, within that year, . . . if you get to know your kids from the beginning, you can help them in so many different ways, and they'll help you, too."

- Think of some times when your accurate understanding of what a student needed positively influenced the effectiveness of your teaching practice.

Chapter Five

Cultivating Positive Relationships With Students

The exemplary teachers clearly expressed that their knowledge of each student supported their ability to teach them effectively. For example, this information made it easier to identify and address student gaps in understanding (see Chapter 4). In this chapter, the exemplary teachers explain their rationale for investing time and energy in ongoing cultivation of positive teacher–student relationships, how this positive quality serves as the foundation of classroom life, and why it pays dividends throughout the year.

- To make this chapter more personally meaningful, think of someone with whom you have a positive relationship. How might you describe what it is like when you are with that person? How does that relationship influence you and your life?

TEACHING AS A SOCIAL ENCOUNTER

Gregory and Gregory identify aspects of teaching as a social encounter, emphasizing the fact that humans are a social species. They highlight how, the moment a human sees another human, instantaneous judgments occur to ascertain the other person's intent and ethical nature.[1] What we each think we know about the other person affects how we decide to behave with them. This naturally arising process occurs for both people throughout each interaction.[2]

Jillian spoke about the link between the quality of teacher–student relationships and learning behavior. She went on to describe how her positive relationships with her students informs their decision-making when learning:

> I think the closer you are to a student, [the more they are] able to feel more confident to ask you questions if they need help. . . . [For example] as the year goes on, I [have] more and more kids feel more comfortable coming up and saying, "I really didn't understand that lesson" or "I need help with my project"—whereas in the beginning of the year, [when] you are still developing your relationships, they might not feel confident in saying that. So, as the year goes on and they are more comfortable with you and they know you are on their side, they will begin to ask more questions and trust in you, too.

Jillian's descriptions relate to Schwartz's discussion of presence in *Connected Teaching*:

> Presence conveys a basic level of acceptance, not necessarily agreement or alignment but more basic human receiving, a momentary commitment to *be with* the other. This acceptance communicates mattering or worth that then potentially helps the other feel less alone and also safe enough to share thinking, ask questions, express concerns, and play with ideas. An intellectually safe space (meaning a space where one can try ideas without fear of ridicule or shame and yet feel motivated by challenge and expectations) is foundational for teaching and learning.[3]

Suzy's comments, though similar to Jillian's and Schwartz's, punctuated the crucial role teacher–student trust plays in education. To Suzy, it is a prerequisite for learning:

> It boils down to trust. Do they trust you? Have you established trust with them? Have you earned their trust? That's it. They *have to* trust you; otherwise, anything you say is meaningless. [Teachers] can talk about valuing [a student's] opinion and showing respect and listening and [when talking] one on one . . . getting down with them on their level, like the same-height chair.
>
> But, it's trust because, if they don't trust you, they don't care what you have to say. And, they are not going to share [anything] with you. . . . Whether it's math or writing or reading, they have to know that you respect them, that you appreciate them, and that you trust them. I think it just all boils down to that one word. . . .
>
> [With trust students think,] "I am not afraid of you. And I know I can say, 'Well, I really wanted to [write] this, but I just didn't know how.'" . . . [The

student is] admitting, "I am vulnerable, but I trust you. And I trust that you're going to help me through this."

Walker similarly articulates the quality of connection in teacher–student(s) relationships: "to experience connection is to participate in a relationship that invites exposure, curiosity, and openness to possibility. Simply put, connection [in positive learning relationships] provides safety from contempt and humiliation; however it does not promise comfort."[4]

- How does the nature of the teacher–student relationship affect your students' learning?

According to Gregory and Gregory, notions of caring, fairness, and concern are ethical elements in educational settings. If students consider their teacher unethical, then that educator's other strengths become less valuable.[5] The teacher's ethical nature influences the part of the self the student shows in the teacher–student relationship and the part the student chooses to share with others in the classroom.

- What connections, if any, can you make between what you have just read and your experience with Part II's "Two Scenarios About Crossing a Room"?
- What comes to mind when you consider Gregory and Gregory's notion of teaching as a social encounter?

MOTIVATION, MEANING, AND FULL ENGAGEMENT

The exemplary teachers spoke of how incredibly hard students will work if they have a strong bond with their teacher. This influential relationship affects the degree to which a student chooses to put forth effort, stretch, struggle, fail, and try again. Rachel highlighted the way her positive teacher–student connections influence student motivation, engagement, and educational outcomes:

> I think it makes them trust you, and if they can trust you, they're going to work for you, they are going to want to . . . make you happy. They're going to want to make you proud. They're going to want to try.
>
> So, just having that connection, building that connection, as soon you can, I think makes a world of a difference for the rest of the year—the outcome, the progress they make—because if they like you and they want to do well for

you, they're going to work hard and try. Even if they struggle, they're going to try, and that's all you can ask from a [student], . . . that they're going to try.

- Think of some specific examples of when your relationship with students affected their interest in learning?

Suzy explained how her commitment to fostering positive relationships serves as the foundation of the learning experience she provides and how it influences authentic student engagement:

> It all starts when they walk in that door, . . . the way you greet them and the way they know that they are coming into your room and they are respected. And they are valued. . . . They are appreciated. And you are the biggest cheerleader for them. And you will not let them give anything less than their best. And it is okay to fail in here because failures are just—hey, that's how we learn.
>
> You know, I think establishing that groundwork, it is so vitally important because otherwise this stuff can be meaningless and boring. But . . . when they know that you are their champion and you really are in their corner, you know what happens? They want to please you. And they really, they buy into this.

Suzy works hard to make learning meaningful for her students so they understand why she is asking them to do a task. Her explicit focus on the meaningfulness of what she requires of her students, combined with the positive quality of their relationship, influences each student's behavioral decision-making when learning.

Patty also spoke about student motivation when learning: "[Students] need to want to do the best they can." Jacobs agrees, stating teachers and schools "choose the [curriculum] path, but ultimately it is the students who determine how they will, or if they can, take steps on the path with each class, each teacher, and each day."[6]

Although, to an observer, some student behavior in the classroom may look the same, there is a difference between a student who is authentically engaged in a learning task and a student who is passively compliant but not actively engaged in learning.[7] According to Bransford, Brown, Cocking, Kober, and others, students need to assimilate new information within their own existing knowledge base when learning.

Knowledge is individually created in each person. It arises from consideration of the ways what is already known might fit with what is being offered in the educational experience. Stated another way, knowledge is known by the knower. It is individually constructed. Therefore, teaching is a knowledge-creating endeavor that results in the learner rearranging and discarding old ideas as a result of more resonant, individually derived understandings.[8]

According to Style, "academic knowledge needs to be seen in relation to the human experience already present in the classroom rather than as something apart from it."[9] If teachers do not know their students well and the academic content lacks connection to their personal background, goals, or interests, then students "can develop an attitude that school is all about other people's agendas—and [the teacher will then] fail to tap [the students'] inner reservoir of motivation and engagement. On the other hand, attuned teachers can use students' intrinsic interest to excite them about what they are learning."[10]

Kytle suggests teachers offer learning opportunities imbued with as many chances as possible for student connections, through as many aspects of who each student is, to solidify, deepen, and sustain learning; this approach will more likely foster focused attention—a deep-learning prerequisite.[11] The ongoing nurturing of positive teacher–student relationships supports an educator's ability to make new content personally relevant, influencing the students' intrinsic motivation, level of engagement, and desire to do their best when learning.

Patty described how she, too, wants to do the best she can for her students. Her conscious awareness of the importance and power of the teaching role is apparent:

> [I] want to build them up so that they can acquire as much as they can while they are [with me], . . . so I basically . . . challenge myself to always be looking for what can I do differently . . . for that [student] or for the whole group. . . . Just make this more exciting, make it more valuable to them, so that they are going to walk away with a set of skills that they need.

- Think back over some of your most successful teaching experiences. What do you think are some of the most influential variables that affected your positive educational outcomes?

NOTICING STUDENT PROGRESS

Effort matters to these educators; it is celebrated. The teachers are on the lookout for and highly value student progress. They know well where their students began academically, and because they intentionally tend to the teacher–student relationship, even small gains become apparent.

Noticing student progress—when the metaphorical light bulb goes on and student understanding is achieved—provides teachers with a deeply felt energy boost when immersed in the challenging work of teaching. Savoring student progress helps support the teacher's sense of efficacy and nurtures the positive teacher–student connection. Both student and teacher have a learning success story that they worked hard to create together. Further sharing the progress with colleagues and parents or caregivers offers more opportunities to relive the positive experience, thereby spreading positivity. It also helps the success stay in memory.[12]

- Think of some times when you have seen a student struggle, persevere, and then learn. What was that experience like for you? What do think your student thought and felt? Consider what role you had in the student's success.
- In what ways have positive teacher–student relationships affected your effort when teaching and your students' effort when learning?

To Katherine, highlighting progress supports development of the students' love of learning. When the teacher points out the progress to the student by explicitly tying those gains to the student's effort and perseverance, it provides the student with clear evidence that hard work creates positive results when learning. People are more likely to experience mistakes as opportunities that serve as a map for growth and development if they have a growth mind-set and believe effort can affect their abilities.[13]

In her teacher–student exchanges, Katherine strives to identify the value of engaging in difficult challenges. She intentionally supports her students' understanding and appreciation of their movement from not knowing to knowing something. She said, "I feel like I am teaching . . . a love of learning. I want them to be invested. I want them to feel like they are learning, . . . [becoming] an improved self, . . . [really seeing all] the little steps . . . that they make. You really have to remind them [of what] they've done."

Katherine intentionally points out what they've learned and the positive consequences of that hard work, drawing students' attention to the specific skills they used to achieve success. She emphasizes what they now can do. For example, after Katherine highlights a student's successful effort learning a number of tricky words, the student may say to her with pride, "'I can read that [now]—it's the word *the*.' And, [Katherine will say], 'Yes you can. See? You did it. . . . You learned it. So that means, that on this page, when you [look] at [the] words, you'll be able to find that word, . . . and if you look even [more] closely, you'll be able to see that you can read other words, too.'"

- What are some ways you nurture your students' love of learning?

The teachers have established different systems and processes so students can follow their improvement as individuals, such as private booklets containing tables that the student fills in to track learning, or on the whole-class level via progress markers on bulletin boards in or near the classroom. Whatever the form, the teachers emphasize the importance of working hard when learning, persevering through difficulties, and creating high-quality work.

- What systems and processes do you use to help students understand and track their improvement?

VALUING SHORT CONVERSATIONS

One way some teachers develop positive relationships with students is by taking the time for short, informal conversations with students about things not necessarily focused on academics and school. Deborah said, "[It's relating] to them. It's talking to them. [For example,] . . . every single day, I am in the hallway greeting them when they come in. Every single day, . . . I get so much information—just out of [that] quick check-in in the morning. . . . I can see how my whole day is going to go, just by the way they come down the hallway." To Kim, "little conversations [communicate to students that] you see them as more than just the student; you see them as a person."

- Why might it matter that students know that their teacher sees them "as a person"?

Over time, these short, informal conversations can provide the teacher with insight into the student's personality, strengths, and way of being. They help the educator make better-informed and more accurate determinations of the student's needs throughout the day. Also, thoughtful identification and leverage of students' strengths when learning has the potential to increase students' energy and interest.[14]

In addition, Kim has found, by listening carefully, she can uncover information in these little conversations that sometimes becomes a valuable teaching tool. For example, if a student is struggling with a math concept, Kim might frame her individualized reteaching of the concept around some aspect of a student's favorite hobby or interest, such as soccer or turtles.

- What might it be like for a student struggling with a tricky academic concept when the teacher reteaches it one on one using an example that includes a favorite hobby?
- What are some ways you identify and use student strengths and interests in your teaching practice?

TIME SAVER

Upper-grade educator Rachel spoke about how cultivating positive relationships through one-on-one conversations with students serves as the foundation of her success. She described how it demonstrates that she cares; makes her interventions with students more successful; and, importantly, saves precious teaching time. She shared an example of what she tends to do when she suspects that something may be off with a student:

> I talk to the [student], if [I've] noticed something is up. I ask them right away. . . . I think if I just watch them for too long, it wastes time, and it's not going to be helpful for them, and I'm going to get frustrated with them, and they're going to get frustrated with whatever I am doing. So that communication piece [is important].
>
> I'll ask them [things like], "What's going on?" "What's up?" "Are you okay?" "Did something happen?" "Why are you upset?" or "Why are you frustrated?" . . . and asking them [one or more of] those questions [and] just repeating questions [to try to understand] I think is really helpful to me . . . because it doesn't waste any time. . . .
>
> I [want] that connection with [my students]. . . . [If] I don't know how to help them, I need to ask them what they need. . . . [Is it] because they are confused, or they're sad, or something happened at home? I can't just help them, without asking them what it is because if it is something at home, it's a totally different conversation than if they are struggling with learning how to divide fractions.
>
> I can help with anything they need . . . [or figure out] who can help them. But until I know what exactly it is, [the student] won't be able to move on, or they won't be able to understand [what I am teaching] or feel like I care about

them. . . . I think it's important to make sure kids know that you do care about them, and by asking those questions, I think it makes them feel more comfortable with me and know that they can trust me.

- Think of some strategies you tend to use in order to determine what your students need?
- How has investing time in cultivating positive teacher–student relationships ended up saving you time?

Deborah discussed how her positive relationships help her more quickly and more accurately understand how and why her students behave the way they do. For example, some students are really sluggish, or they may exhibit other behaviors on Monday mornings. She knows, for some of those students, the reason is "they are hungry" after a weekend at home, so she gives them food before asking them to do anything else.

RESPECT, MUTUALITY, HARD WORK, AND ENERGY

Relationships form and are maintained through the contributions of each person in the relationship. The educator's social-emotional skill set—self-awareness, self-management, social awareness, relationship skills, and responsible decision-making—affects how each teacher–student relationship develops.[15]

To Katherine and Suzy, their deliberately respectful attitude serves as the core of their approach to nurturing positive relationships. Katherine spoke about the intentionality of her contributions to her teacher–student relationships. She said that part of her "role as a teacher is to show [my students] that I respect them *greatly*. . . . I think . . . when you put something out, you get it back." Suzy also described her contribution to her relationships with students: "If I want them to give me their best, I have to earn . . . their respect and their appreciation and their trust."

- What are some ways you communicate your respect for your students?
- What are some ways you earn your students "respect and their appreciation and their trust"?

Some of the teachers spoke about how their positive connections with students served as an important source of energy throughout the day. Four of the educators characterized the positive energy exchange in these relationships as feeding off each other. For example, Deborah said, "I feed off [their energy], too. . . . It's a give and take. . . . As I give them, they give back to me."

These comments relate to Wellesley College's Jean Baker Miller's ideas that help explain the power of positive relationships to foster human growth and development.[16] According to Miller, mutually positive, growth-fostering relationships are characterized by *five good things* for each person:

1. A sense of zest that arises from the connection
2. An enhanced motivation and ability to act within and outside of the relationship
3. Increased knowledge of the self and other(s) in the relationship
4. An increased desire for more relational connections
5. Greater self-worth [17]

- In what ways do you think positive teacher–student relationships support your students' ability to bring their best to their learning?

Some teachers highlighted aspects of mutuality in their teacher–student relationships. For example, Deborah said, "We work hard. I work hard. My kids work hard." There is energy and power in the dynamic of shared teacher–student priorities and everyone's hard work. The shared effort has meaning and purpose. Barb said, "I'm tired at the end of the day. And you know . . . it's a good feeling to be tired at the end of the day. If I'm not tired at the end of the day, then I don't feel like I've given all I need to give [to my students]."

- Think of times when you have worked hard on something you found deeply meaningful. How would you describe the experience? What made it so meaningful to you?
- In what ways might Deborah's and Barb's teacher–student relationships influence their experience of their work?

To Rachel, the cultivation of positive teacher–student relationships is a high priority. She suggests teachers

> build those relationships as soon as you can . . . because the stronger they get, . . . the better it's going to be for everybody. . . . [It's] even [for] my wellbeing, [too]. Those relationships at school [are key]. I mean you're going

into work every day; you need to have those positive relationships. If you don't, work's not going to be fun, the job's not going to be fun, teaching's not going to be fun, [and] the kids are going to suffer.

Taxer, Becker-Kurz, and Frenzel agree: "high quality teacher–student relationships help protect teachers from being emotionally exhausted through increasing the amount of enjoyment and decreasing the amount of anger they experience in the classroom."[18]

- Think of some examples when your positive relationships with students enhanced your enjoyment of teaching. In what ways did it affect your level of energy?
- What are some approaches you use to develop high-quality relationships with your students?

Chapter Six

Negotiating Difficult Relationships With Students

While the exemplary teachers agreed about the importance of developing positive relationships with students, some educators highlighted times when they found connecting with a student quite difficult. Personality clashes can occur. Rachel said, sometimes students just "get along better with the other teacher and not me, [or] the opposite [can happen, too]." Not all teacher–student relationships evolve smoothly or easily. This chapter explores how the exemplary teachers negotiate difficult relationships and its influence on their teaching success.

- Think of a time when you had a complicated relationship with a student. What specific aspects of your social and emotional skill set—the five core competencies of self-awareness, self-management, social awareness, relationship skills, and responsible decision-making—supported your success?[1]
- How were you able to negotiate the difficulties?

Negative teacher–pupil relationships not only affect students, but they influence teachers, as well.[2] A teacher's memory of a difficult exchange with a challenging student potentially cues a teacher's negative emotional response whenever that student enters the classroom.[3] This memory imbued with negative emotion can also seep into interactions with the student's family members.

Research suggests challenging relationships with students can foster negative teacher emotions that, if experienced chronically, adversely affect teacher motivation, reduce teaching quality, and enhance teacher burnout.[4] Conversely, Frymier and Houseer assert higher levels of student motivation and learning occur when the relationship between teacher and student is a positive one.[5]

- What tools do you currently use to support your resilience when negotiating a difficult relationship?

VALUES, CONNECTIONS, AND ASKING FOR HELP

According to Cullen and Brito Pons, researchers have found that willpower strengthens, stress reduces, openness increases, and bias decreases when people consider, clarify, and prioritize their values.[6] Katie shared how staying grounded in her values of treating students with respect, kindness, and fairness supports her ability to negotiate difficult relationships:

> I think just being respectful to each other is huge because I think [if] kids know . . . you're kind and you're fair, that's . . . everything. Because if they don't think you are fair . . . and they don't think you like them, then you've lost them. You know what I mean? . . . So, yeah, relationships are first and foremost. They can't learn if they don't feel that you like them and have their back and treat them well. If you don't give respect, the kids are not going to give respect in return, and it's just going to be an awful year. So, you've just got to connect with everybody.

- What values, beliefs, and principles guide your life, in general, and inform your interactions with others, more specifically?

While it is clear from her comments that Deborah agrees with Katie's sentiments, Deborah also shared how challenging it can be sometimes to find and nurture a teacher–student connection: "If I know I am not clicking with somebody, I try to find a way to make that click. . . . There's always something that you can connect with, but it's a matter of finding it, and not everybody's going to give it to you as easily; some you really have to work for." With one student, Deborah ultimately found a connection when she learned that he enjoyed having a pet snake. Although she "can't stand snakes," Deborah does have a dog that she loves. Deborah ended up using this mutual interest and love of their pets as the basis of their informal conversations, thereby enhancing their teacher–student connection and influencing the quality of their relationship.

- Have you ever had a difficult time connecting with a student? If so, what did you do?

University of Pittsburgh's H. Richard Milner offers the following five suggestions for nurturing teacher–student connections:

1. Interview your students. . . .
2. Give assignments that allow students to share their experiences and interests. . . .
3. Encourage classroom discussions that let students be the center of attention. . . .
4. Attend extracurricular activities featuring your students. . . .
5. Visit a site in your students' community.[7]

The breadth of student needs in classrooms today can make the negotiation of teacher–student relationships challenging.[8] Rachel emphasized how one of the most important keys to her success was her comfort with reaching out and asking for help from colleagues, administrators, and parents and caregivers to find ways to connect with and best support students:

> There are certain kids that come into your classroom that maybe their behavior is not something you have ever worked with before. And you are not prepared. I mean, I'm not a psychologist, so I have no idea how to work with kids that have those emotional or behavioral disabilities and/or . . . just issues or whatever it is [students are struggling with], so, you just have to learn to work with it. . . . Once you see it, [you need to] figure out a way to work with it because you're going to have it. . . . You [just] have to figure out how to make it work.

- Who are some people you tend to reach out to for support?
- What are some consequences that can occur when the teacher–student connection is lacking? How can it affect the teacher? How can it affect the student? What are the ways it influences teaching and learning in the classroom?

WHAT WE NOTICE AND WHAT WE MISS

As mentioned in Chapter 2, human perception is limited.[9] People cannot see what occurs outside their narrow focus of attention.[10] We each have influential expectations that inform what we notice and how we interpret it.[11] Our expectations also affect what we miss.[12] To complicate matters, confirmation bias makes what we already think, feel, and believe more relevant to notice.[13]

Barb highlighted the influence of teacher expectations, the power teachers wield, and the significance of the challenge when a teacher–student relationship becomes markedly negative:

> I think [it's the] teacher's job . . . to get the best out of each child and the child gets the best out of you. . . . As a teacher, I'm always learning from them, and I'm going and digging . . . in my bag of tricks to figure out what's going to work for [each of them]. . . . I think [teacher expectations play] a huge role, and I think it can make or break [each student]. And I hate to say [it], but we . . . have a powerful role in these [students'] lives, and we spend a lot of time with them, . . . and it's really sad when it's not working well.

One feature hardwired into human perception systems that can exacerbate the situation is our tendency to notice what is wrong and negative.[14] As researchers Baumeister, Bratslavsky, Finkenauer, and Vohs state, "bad is stronger than good."[15] This negativity bias causes the negative in situations to stand out, so it is noticed more readily. In addition, negative experiences are more easily remembered and can be more vividly relived than positive.[16] We can see this negativity bias tendency in ourselves when considering our interest in the news. Negative news tends to grab our attention in a different way than positive news. This important brain wiring supported our survival as a species.[17]

Another complicating factor affecting the negotiation of difficult teacher–student relationships is our capacity to miss positive student behavior, even if the student is right in front of us. As Appiah states, "It's easy to miss something you are not looking for."[18] Because we cannot take in everything there is to see, other aspects of the environment, which we already believe are important to notice and pay attention to, tend to take precedence.[19]

- What comes to mind when you consider the ways that teacher expectations, confirmation bias, and negativity bias affect teacher–student relationships and the development of student reputations?

Importantly, researchers have found people tend to mistakenly believe that they *will definitely* notice distinctive or unusual features in a situation, but in actuality, these often remain unnoticed.[20] Although it may seem implausible, human perception is an incomplete process that feels comprehensive, accurate, and complete.[21]

- Have you ever become aware that you missed something that occurred right in front of you?

Should you want to experience this sometimes-surprising aspect of human perception, please see the links to information and experiments in appendix F listed under Inattentional Blindness, Change Blindness, and Selective Attention.

- In what ways might the incomplete nature of human perception contribute to the continuance of difficult teacher–student relationships?

SEEING BEYOND THE MORE OBVIOUS NEGATIVE

The teacher's perception of and relationship with each student affects the educator's ability to identify and nurture the best that each student has to offer.[22] Teacher decision-making (e.g., to explain, paraphrase, redirect, reprimand, encourage) is a function of teacher focusing, noticing, interpreting, and ultimately deciding. Each decision is informed by how the teacher perceives the student and the corresponding nature of the teacher–student relationship.

 Katherine shared an example of a time when other adults in the building who didn't know one of her students very well would say things to her like "He's really fresh" or "He's very disrespectful." Her student had a different relationship with those adults, and he, as a result, behaved somewhat differently with them than with her. Katherine went on to explain, saying with a small smile,

> I know that he *can* have [that] effect on people. . . . But, it also can be a defense mechanism, where, when you know the [student] better and you get to know them, then you . . . [see] there is that surface of the behavior.
>
> But then, when you see them working and you kind of connect with them on a more, you know, emotional level, you see what they are capable of—what they try when they realize that they are safe, and . . . they can trust you. You . . . see a [student] in a different light.

Katherine believes that there is more to her student than initially meets the eye. She also believes there are underlying reasons for a student's behavior. She understands that people have many different aspects of who they are, and she appreciates the ways the relationship and the context, among other variables, play a role in influencing what aspect emerges. Katherine presupposes that positives in her student are worth seeking and finding. These presuppositions influence what Katherine sees, thinks, and feels when looking at a student and what she contributes to the teacher–student relationship. Katherine trusts that her efforts to forge a positive relationship will help support students' abilities and willingness to share the best of what they have to offer.

- How do your presuppositions influence what you see, think, and feel when looking at a student?
- What contributes to your ability to "see a student in a different light"?
- To make the following exploration of relationships more personally relevant, think about what happens to you the moment you see someone you think may not like you. In that moment, what do you think and feel? How does it affect your behavioral decision-making? What part of yourself is amplified when you are with that person? What do you tend to contribute to that relationship?

In every teacher–student exchange, each person's perceptions have a powerful role to play in what aspects of themselves and the other arise.[23] The relationship is cocreated, in part, through what each person thinks is important to notice about the other person. Surrey and Kramer explain that we are "interactive and interreactive creatures; conditioned reactivity in one triggers the patterns of reactivity in the other, impacting and influencing each other in an ongoing dance of interreactivity."[24]

In other words, the teacher and the student simultaneously contribute to the relationship. Moment by moment, beliefs and expectations affect what each person notices, how that information is understood, and what emotion arises. Emotion plays an important role. Negative emotion narrows perception processes, while positive emotion broadens them.[25] Emotion and perception are further explored in the next chapter.

- Think of a time when you intentionally altered what you were contributing to a relationship. What did you do? What happened? What helped?

According to Margaret Cullen, a Stanford University School of Medicine Center for Compassion and Altruism Research and Education (CCARE) trainer, compassion skill development can support a teacher's ability to alter entrenched negative teacher–student relationships. After training with Cullen, teachers reported they no longer found the need to seek evidence of how difficult some students were to solidify their cases against them.[26]

When considering Cullen's outcomes, it can be helpful to remember that human perception is limited.[27] Moment by moment, we each make conscious and unconscious decisions about what is important to notice, thereby affecting where we focus our attention. As mentioned previously, we cannot take in everything, even if it is right in front of us.

Over time, the teachers' experiences with a variety of Cullen's compassion practices allowed a greater variety of information about their students to emerge. This influenced each teachers' sense of situation and the student. With training, the educators found they were able to release their habitual and narrow focus of finding evidence of the students' negative behavior. Instead, they began to see evidence of the students' positive behavior, too.[28]

- How might the broadened perception of the student and the situation have influenced what each teacher contributed to their relationships with their students?

In *The Mindfulness-Based Emotional Balance Workbook*, Cullen and Brito Pons share ideas and exercises related to self-awareness, compassion, thought-feeling awareness, mindfulness, and forgiveness as vehicles for negotiating difficult situations.[29]

- Consider a time when you needed to negotiate a difficult relationship with a student. In what ways did your perception of the student inform your decision-making process? What skills, strengths, and approaches supported your success?

For more about compassion and other contemplative practices, please see the research-based information and exercises listed under Mindfulness, Compassion, and Gratitude in appendix F.

SELF-AWARENESS, MINDFULNESS, AND AN ANNOYING STUDENT

Kayla described how, a number of years ago, she had a student who *really* "rubbed [her] the wrong way." She explained how she still couldn't clearly explain or identify why she had such an automatic negative response to the student, but her negative response was quite strong. Recognizing her annoyance with the student's natural way of being, she worked hard to be extremely mindful whenever she spoke to him during the year.

Kayla closely monitored her responses to him and chose to be effusively positive whenever possible. The situation required a tremendous amount of self-awareness and self-management. Kayla said, "I tried *so hard* to not let him see that, just [his] little mannerisms really, were getting to me. (pause) . . . I can't let this [student] know that there is something that is just not clicking with me." She knew what she contributed to their relationship would be highly influential.

Looking back, she wondered if maybe she had overdone it with the abundance of positive remarks. However, years later, the student told Kayla that she was his favorite teacher. This was especially significant for her because of how cognizant she had to be of her response to him every day. Kayla described how she did not want her annoyance with this student's natural manner to cause him to "hate school" and negatively affect his life.

- What are some ways you manage strong feelings about students?

Contemplative practice is one way to support greater overall awareness, lessen reactivity, and enhance self-awareness.[30] Through consistent use, it can uncover and provide insight into current habits of perception. For example, enhanced mindfulness can make the raw material culled from a situation more apparent. It also can help illuminate how what has been noticed is interpreted.

Smalley and Winston of the Mindful Awareness Research Center (MARC) at the University of California, Los Angeles, describe mindfulness as a "means of seeing the conceptual frameworks by which you live—how your thoughts shape your worldview." They go on to explain, "The body of knowledge you accumulate, your thoughts, your interactions, memories, and experiences, all shape and reshape your worldview, which is the lens through which you filter your experience. Mindfulness is a means of investigating such frameworks—your belief systems, your biases, your blind spots."[31]

Stated another way, mindfulness practices can enhance understanding of what you notice and how you make sense of what you notice. Salzberg describes mindfulness as a "relational quality, in that it does not depend on what is happening. [It is instead] about how [you] are relating to what is happening."[32]

- What do you do in order to gain insight into how you are relating to what is happening?

In addition to enhancing an ability to relax, various mindfulness practices can support a deepened awareness of perception habits and tendencies, such as the placement and focus of attention, your inner dialogue, your judgments, and what you use as the basis of determinations concerning what is happening and what is possible. Importantly, there is emerging research that suggests the consistent use of mindfulness practices can positively influence educators in a variety of ways, such as reducing their stress and burnout, enhancing their emotional competence, and improving their classroom practices.[33]

Students also benefit from learning mindfulness skills.[34] According to Scheberlein and Sheth, "when teachers are fully present, they teach better. When students are fully present, the quality of their learning is better."[35]

- What inhibits and what supports your ability to be focused and fully present when teaching?
- What helps you relax and recharge?

REMEMBERING THE ROLE'S POWER AND INFLUENCE

Kim's awareness of how much positive power she wields supports her ability to negotiate challenges with students. She shared some examples involving students who are in the foster care system:

> You know it's not the greatest relationship that they have with the foster parent. So, they come in, and they are having a bad day. And I'm there for the

hugs, you know. . . . It goes back to the trust and [students] knowing that they have someone that they can . . . count on. . . . It might not be the person at home, but they know they can come here every day, and there's a consistent person who will *always* be here for them.

That's why I feel it is so important that, at the end of each day, . . . regardless [of] how crummy a day someone might have had, [that students] know when they come in tomorrow, that's all forgotten. . . . We are starting fresh.

Kim knows she has the power to positively affect her students' lives. This understanding informs her rationale to try to appreciate the broad range of contributing factors that affect students' behavior. Being open to and curious about the small, medium, and large factors in play supports her understanding of what is happening with her students and why.[36] Kim's emotional agility, brought about by, among other things, her self-awareness and self-management skills, supports her ability to handle the situation and then provide the student with the chance to start fresh after a "crummy" day.

- How are you able to handle difficult situations with equanimity?

According to Susan David, author of *Emotional Agility*, "emotionally agile people are not immune to stresses and setbacks. The key difference is they know how to gain critical insight about situations and interactions from their feelings, and use this knowledge to adapt, align their values and actions, and make changes to bring the best of themselves forward."[37]

- Think about the attributes and talents you bring to your teaching practice. What is it about you that supports your ability to manage your emotions in the moment, when a student is having a "crummy" day?
- What do you do that helps you set difficult experiences aside and move on with authentic openness and positivity?

Chapter Seven

Investing in a Positive Learning Environment

Because we are a social species, relational and cultural variables are in play whenever we gather together. As mentioned previously, we influence and are affected by other individuals; we are also affected by cultural norms and group dynamics.[1]

- Consider some examples from your own life to test this out. Think of some group experiences you would identify as positive and productive. Now think of some less than positive and productive group experiences. What do you think are some of the key factors differentiating the two?
- From your experience, what does a positive and productive classroom look like, sound like, and feel like?

In this chapter, the exemplary teachers share how and why they invest time and energy into developing a positive and productive learning environment. The exploration begins with Barb's summary of key environmental aspects that she strives to create:

> Each day is positive, reflective, [and] supportive. . . . [Students] know their role . . . in the classroom, . . . [and I have very] high expectations for each and every [student] that enters my room. . . . They're accountable. . . . [In here] there's movement, there's talking, [and] there's a lot of support. . . . They [also] know that I care. They know that I'm going to be there for them. . . . That's the atmosphere.

- How might you describe the atmosphere you strive to create in your classroom?

According to the National Academies of Sciences consensus study concerning effective instruction and the classroom environment,

> Effective instruction depends on understanding [the] complex interplay among students' prior knowledge, experiences, motivations, interests, language, and cognitive skills and the cultural, social, cognitive, and emotional characteristics of the learning environment. When challenging work is coupled with high expectations and high levels of support, and when students are actively working and cognitively, socially, and emotionally engaged, this produces greater motivation, stronger identity development, and deeper learning.[2]

RELATIONSHIPS AND LEARNING

Gone are the mostly silent classrooms where teachers do a majority of the talking, desks face forward in neat rows, and students sit in seats filling out a series of workbooks. Classrooms today require interaction. The nature and quality of student–student relationships affect learning outcomes. Each student's social and emotional skill set—identified as the five core competencies of self-awareness, self-management, social awareness, relationships skills, and responsible decision-making—influences classroom interactions throughout each day.[3]

Teacher social-emotional learning (SEL) also plays a powerful role in educational outcomes.[4] Jones, Bouffard, and Weissbourd explain,

> Teachers' SEL competencies influence students in at least three ways. . . . First, [it affects] the quality of teacher–student relationships. . . . Second, teachers model SEL skills for students—intentionally or not. Teachers navigate stressful situations nearly every day, and students are watching. . . . Third, teachers' SEL abilities likely influence their classroom organization and management.[5]

The Collaborative for Academic, Social, and Emotional Learning (CASEL) identify adult and student social and emotional learning as a "powerful lever for creating caring, just, inclusive, and healthy communities that support all individuals in reaching their fullest potential."[6]

As Suzy highlighted in chapter 1, teaching is an "incredibly challenging job, and it is becoming more challenging with every year, [with] the dynamics of children that are coming in with their *exceptionally* diverse needs." The educators in the study work hard to create the best possible learning environment for all. Their rationale aligns with the research findings shared in *The Brain Basis for Integrated Social, Emotional, and Academic Development: How Emotions and Social Relationships Drive Learning.*[7]

For example, Rachel places a high value on her students being kind and supportive of one another. She said, "Teaching [students] how to be good people . . . and classmates, I think, is really important. . . . I think strong relationships . . . make for a better classroom environment."

- What are some ways you teach students how to be good people and classmates?
- How do you nurture student–student relationships in order to support development of a positive learning environment?

Kim intentionally and explicitly values the students' role in helping support everyone's learning:

> We all help each other. . . . I love to make an example out of somebody who says something differently than I did and somebody else has an *ah-ha* moment because of [what their classmate said]. I have them share that with the class. Or [I will sometimes] have the other person who learned something say what their [classmate] shared [that was helpful]. . . . The [students] need to see each other as . . . resources to understand they're valuable. Not just . . . being a friend [to each other], but [they can actively be] helping [one another] with their learning, [as well].

- In what ways can seeing each other as resources influence student–student relationships, in general, and learning when students are working in pairs or small groups?

Suzy referred to the role of culture in the day-to-day life of the classroom community. Culture informs each person's way of seeing, interpreting, and being in the world.[8] Berman, Chaffee, and Sarmiento describe how "open conversations about culture and cultural experiences teach students to appreciate the perspective of others and the richness that diversity brings to learning."[9] Suzy views cultural understanding as a vital skill set her students will need to use throughout their lifetime:

[Each] of our cultures matters, and our traditions matter, and our heritage matters. It builds [our identity]—who we are. . . . [Students] need to know [about culture] in this world that we live in. We have got to respect each other, and one way we do that is by listening to each other, and sharing. . . . We can't be afraid to share [ourselves with one another].

- In your experience, how does a learning environment influence how a student feels about sharing?
- In what ways is your classroom's culture similar to and different from your students' home culture?

Gaitan stresses the importance of teacher inquiry into whose culture is supported in the learning environment. For example, in what ways do students need to alter their natural, organic way of being and functioning in order to succeed in the classroom setting? *Cultural continuity* is a term Gaitan uses when referring to school experiences that are consistent with those from the student's home culture. Students who experience cultural continuity are at an advantage because it is easier for them to take in new information when the cultural context does not also need to be negotiated.[10]

- How might cultural continuity influence the students in your classroom?
- Consider a time when you were in a group situation where people in the group had a different culture than your own. It may be interesting to note how, in big and small ways, your thoughts and feelings and, ultimately, your behavior in that group was influenced by the cultural difference.
- Now consider a group situation where people had a similar culture to yours. Think about how, in big and small ways, your thoughts and feelings and, ultimately, your behavior in that group was influenced by the group's cultural familiarity.
- What did you notice when reflecting about yourself in these different scenarios? What connections come to mind when you think about present or past students' experiences?

CLARITY AND CONSISTENCY

Though they manage their classrooms using different processes and varied techniques, nearly all of the exemplary practitioners at some point brought up the importance of having an organized, predictable, positive classroom environment with clear procedures, plans, structures, routines, roles, and responsibilities. This context supports the educator's ability to teach and the students' ability to learn. June relayed how helpful it is to have a clear sense of what you want to have happen and an awareness of student responses to teacher techniques so precious learning time is not wasted:

> I wouldn't call myself organized, but in here I am! (Laughs) We have the same routines so [the students] know what to do, basically. If I say, "Get your book out. We are going to do this," they know what I am talking about. . . . It's [our] routine. . . .
>
> [As a teacher, it is important to develop a] sense [about] wasted time or time *not* on task and why [it may be happening]. [It's also important to understand] how to manage time on task. . . . [You need to know] what it really looks like. . . . And, just knowing the kids [is key]—you know which ones to zoom in on, . . . [like noticing] the kid that's daydreaming. . . . [You] know who to watch for. . . . [You need to have] clear expectations and [know] who's off task. . . . Having a [clear] vision of what you want your classroom . . . to be like [is so helpful].

- What is your vision? What do you want your classroom to be like?

Patty also discussed how consistency contributes to the foundation of positive and productive learning communities. To Patty, this notion of predictability refers to classroom processes as well as teacher mood and behavior:

> I tell the [students] quite often that [our] rules never change, . . . so [they] never have to worry when [they] come in [that things will be different and they won't know what to do]. . . . I want to create a safe environment, something that [students] are comfortable with. . . . [And, the students] know that they are held responsible for those rules no matter what. I try to be as consistent as possible.
>
> I don't feel like my personality [or mood] interferes—in fluctuating with my day. I [mean] my family at home knows that, when I am here, this is totally my world. I am [focused. I'm] not anywhere else when I am here, so I won't be calling [home] unless there is an emergency. I won't be . . . checking in [with them] or whatever. . . . [They know my total focus at school is teaching]. I separate those worlds as much as I can, so I don't bring it into the classroom. . . . [That's important.] I feel like when I am here, I am pretty even-keeled on a day-to-day basis. I think that [the students] know what to expect, and I like to keep it that way.

- In your experience, what role does a predictable classroom environment (teacher behavior and classroom routines) play in teaching and learning?

Patty and others referenced how nurturing a positive classroom environment fosters student readiness by providing the sense of safety required in order to truly learn. Schonert-Reichl agrees, stating students "who feel comfortable with their teachers and peers are more willing to grapple with challenging material and persist at difficult learning tasks."[11]

Debbie captured this sentiment: "[Students] need to be in a safe spot emotionally and mentally so that they can take the risk." According to Tyng, Amin, Saad, and Malik, "emotion has a substantial influence on the cognitive processes in [people], including perception, attention, learning, memory, reasoning, and problem solving. Emotion has a particularly strong influence on attention. . . . [In short,] emotion modulates virtually every aspect of cognition."[12] Goleman and Senge further highlight how the "brain's centers for learning operate at their peak when [people] are focused and calm. As we become upset, these centers work less well. In the grip of extreme agitation, we can only focus on what's upsetting us and learning shuts down."[13]

- Think of situations from your own experience as a learner when your emotions interfered with your ability to learn something new. What was happening? What helped?
- What have you noticed about your students' emotional state and their capacity to learn?

INVESTING TIME AND CREATING A HIGH-FUNCTIONING CLASSROOM

Jillian's preferred teaching methodology heavily features student collaborations. As mentioned elsewhere, her students work together (pairs, trios, small groups) at least once on every educational task. Student–student relationships are complicated, and Jillian's teaching approach does not work perfectly. However, Jillian has found that her ongoing efforts to nurture a positive learning environment supports productive and fruitful student–student learning. Please see chapters 5 and 6 for additional ideas.

Jillian's approach aligns with Director Patricia Kuhl's research at the University of Washington's National Science Foundation (NSF) Learning in Informal and Formal Environments (LIFE) Center. Kuhl identifies teaching practices that leverage students' social brains, such as face-to-face interactions and small-group work, as central to high-quality learning environments.[14]

Jillian referenced how her ongoing investment in nurturing student–student relationships pays dividends when using this teaching approach. Her knowledge of each student also plays a role in enhancing the success of student pairings and groupings. In addition, for this pedagogy to be successful, Jillian spoke about class management and emphasized the clear establishment and maintenance of positive learning routines and processes:

> You definitely need to set the community, set that early, right away. I think if you have an open [atmosphere], (pause) a place where [students] can take chances and know it's okay to fail and take risks, I think that correlates directly to [your students' behavior], . . . so, if you promote it and *you* show it, in return [the students] are able. [Over time] the community itself changes. . . . They know your drills, they know how it's going to work, so . . . by setting that tone and those expectations [early], . . . they are able to exemplify [your expectations]—what you've said and what you've shown.

- What are some approaches you use to "set the community" in your classroom?

Some teachers spoke about how helpful it is to collaboratively establish community guidelines by cocreating with students achievable classroom norms rather than stating premade teacher-developed rules. The educators find the collaboration promotes greater student investment in the day-to-day functioning of the classroom community.

Katherine described how having a high-functioning group is one of her keys to success; it allows her to carve out one-on-one time with each student. Katherine explained that, in order to do her job well, she needed to

> get to know each and every child. . . . You need to see where they are and where they have to go. . . . You *have* to do it [one-on-one] because you could have a [student] that just flows right through [group work] because they are really verbal, . . . they raise their hand all the time, . . . they participate, and they're happy. . . . [Those students] have this really great way of being a chameleon, and [they can] kind of just . . . [adapt] to the group.
>
> But, when you sit down with them [one-on-one]—it's where you really, (pause) you get to know what they're doing, what they know, what they need to work on, you know? Where are [the] gaps? [My one-on-one] observing and assessing, . . . not necessarily like the assessment that . . . the city throws at you, it's [more informal], (pause) it's "How is it going?" . . . My informal

assessments . . . help me understand where [each] child is and how [to best teach each of them].

As a result, Katherine invests one to two months establishing the classroom's learning environment. Katherine said she focuses on teaching students "how to be as independent as they can [be] . . . how to work together cooperatively . . . how to follow directions. [I want to] make things expected." This high-functioning class dynamic allows Katherine to pull all children aside periodically one-on-one to conduct short, "little snapshot" assessments while the rest of her class works successfully on other things.

During her "little snapshot" assessments, Katherine is trying to ascertain what and how her students are thinking and feeling. We humans have the ability to predict someone's future behavior by, loosely stated, attempting to read someone else's mind. Goleman refers to the notion, theory of mind, to explain our ability to recognize that other people also have an individualized logical framework of perception and understanding.[15]

Medina characterizes theory of mind as, in part, the inferences humans make about the motivations of others. According to Medina, it is vital that teachers strive to know what each of their students are thinking and feeling in order to make effective educational interventions and teach them well.[16]

- What are some strategies you use to try to know what each of your students are thinking and feeling?

An educator's theory of mind affects how the teacher perceives student understanding of lesson content, possible interventions for clarification, and supportive steps for deepening learning.[17] Nichols suggests that teachers appreciate the way their personal cultural norms affect their interpretations of their students' understanding and behavior.[18]

According to Eberhardt, "when something is regarded as a norm, people . . . are not only inclined to believe that the norm is just 'the way things are'; they are inclined to believe that something normative is 'the way things *should* be.'" Enhanced teacher cultural awareness can lead to a more broadly considered and accurate assessment of students' actions and reactions during the educational experience.[19]

For example, the commonly used IRE question-answer cycle, involving teacher-initiated communication (I), student response (R), and teacher evaluation of response (E), has strong cultural components.[20] A teacher may interpret a student's limited participation as evidence of the student's lack of understanding or interest, laziness, shyness, or oppositional behavior, when in fact that student's behavior could be a culturally derived restraint. This might occur if the student's home culture is one where silence is favored over talking, elders are not questioned nor looked at directly, or succinct speech is a sign of maturity.

- Think of examples from your teaching experience where your knowledge about your own and your students' cultural backgrounds influenced the accuracy of your interpretations of your students' behaviors.

TENDING TO GROUP DEVELOPMENT

All the educators put a high value on establishing and maintaining a supportive learning context over the course of the year. Throughout each school day, the intertwined and influential relationships among students, as well as teacher–student relationships, affect learning processes and the overall learning environment.[21] According to Tuckman and Jensen, the intentional tending to a group's development over time can influence how the group grows and changes.[22]

Some teachers described how valuing kindness, humor, or laughter, as well as having fun together, positively affected their group dynamic. Deborah said,

> I love the sense of building a class. . . . We have 180 days together, and I love that sense of like, they own me, and I own them, . . . and we just, enjoy each other, and I *do* think . . . it's okay to stop every once in a while. . . . I say, "We're going to sprinkle in some fun!" . . . You build [your community]. . . . It's a relationship—you work at it, you develop it. . . . Learning is enjoyable, and we have fun together. And it's a win-win.

This orientation to cultivating authentic positivity may be a clue that helps explain the exemplary teachers' educational outcomes. Researchers have found that positive emotions, such as interest, gratitude, inspiration, amusement, pride, joy, serenity, love, awe, and hope, can cause human brain functioning that is broader, less stereotypical, more relational, complex, and creative.[23]

In addition, when people are in a positive emotional state, perception widens, and they process information differently than when they are feeling negative emotion.[24] With positive emotions, Fredrickson has found people have a greater momentary thought-action repertoire, or "range of potential actions the body and mind are prepared to take."[25]

- Think about a time when you were in a negative emotional state. Can you bring to mind how your perception narrowed?
- Now consider an opposite situation—a time when you were in a positive emotional state. Can you remember a broadened perception when you were experiencing that positive emotion? If so, what was that like for you?

Research suggests the experience of a positive emotion supports the development of clearer connections between disparate ideas.[26] Fredrickson further highlights how "the expanded cognitive flexibility evident during positive emotional states results in resource building that becomes useful over time. Even though a positive emotional state can be only momentary, the benefits last in the form of traits, social bonds, and abilities that endure into the future."[27]

Positive emotions also can act as a buffer and enhance resilience. What's more, positive emotions foster an upward spiral of positivity that can spread between and among people[28]; "The implication of [this research] is that positive emotions have inherent value to human growth and development and cultivation of these emotions will help people lead fuller lives."[29]

- Given what you have just read, in what ways can the experience of positive emotions—interest, gratitude, inspiration, amusement, pride, joy, serenity, love, awe, hope—influence educational outcomes in your setting?
- What comes to mind when you consider how teachers can personally benefit from investing in creating and tending to a positive classroom environment?

Chapter Eight

Connecting With Parents and Caregivers

This chapter explores how the exemplary teachers cultivate positive relationships with their students' parents and caregivers and what is gained from those efforts. To begin, Katie stated how highly she values nurturing a positive teacher–parent or –caregiver "connection, to get everyone on the same page. . . . [We need to] be partners in the education process, not, like, separate entities."

- Consider the role your students' parents and caregivers play in your teaching practice.
- What are some ways you connect with your parent and caregiver community?

Positive school–home partnerships can play a key role in teaching success. According to Epstein, Christenson, Reschly, and others, effective educators are knowledgeable about their students' family backgrounds, and they strive to create positive and productive school–family relationships.[1] These relationships, like all connections between people, are affected by each person's expectations, past experiences, and culture (e.g., socioeconomic status, ethnicity, schooling, personality, age, gender, social class, etc.), among other variables.

One cultural variable that can significantly affect the nature of home–school connections is the parent's or caregiver's past schooling experiences. The Collaborative for Academic, Social and Emotional Learning (CASEL) highlights how important it is "to remember that not all families have fond memories of and experiences with schools. In fact, these prior experiences can have a deep impact on how willing families are to pursue partnerships with their child's school."[2]

- What are your thoughts about how cultural similarities (e.g., socioeconomic status, ethnicity, schooling, personality, age, gender, social class, etc.) affect the relationships you make with your students' parents and caregivers?
- How might cultural differences (e.g., socioeconomic status, ethnicity, schooling, personality, age, gender, social class, etc.) affect the relationships you make with your students' parents and caregivers?
- How might cultural similarities, differences, or both influence how each of your students' parents and caregivers see you?

DEVELOPING THE TEACHER–PARENT AND TEACHER–CAREGIVER RELATIONSHIP

While the exemplary teachers want to develop a positive relationship with their students' parents and caregivers, different teachers use different ways to facilitate strong school–home connections. Some examples are letters sent home before the school year begins (written in the student's home language); periodic check-in phone calls; quick informal in-person conversations; invitations to classroom events and celebrations; invitations to share family traditions, stories, and talents; invitations to support the classroom logistics; scheduled one-on-one meetings; and ongoing texts, e-mails, and use of other technology to support timely communications.

Barb's school–home link is a point of pride. It is a high priority, and she works hard to reach out and make connections with her students' parents and caregivers. To Barb, this investment of time and energy pays off. She thinks it is one of the most significant influences on her success as a teacher:

> One of the things I do is . . . write a letter at the beginning of the year to let them know about me, and I ask them, as a family, to write a letter about them and to share that with me, so then I can get an idea . . . of them. . . .
>
> I do a lot of outreach with my parents. I have a website. I do a lot of e-mailing weekly with them, so we're in contact. . . . Even if they don't speak English, I do my translation and all of that. . . . I try to get to know them right [away, right] at the beginning.

[I think] it is a huge link. The link between school and home is [one of] the best [things] you can do to provide success for . . . students. . . . [It] is something that I've prided myself in doing. I've done it since I started teaching. I used to use little books, and I would write notes [that would be brought home and then returned to school]. . . . Now, of course, . . . with e-mailing and all of that, it's much easier. . . . And, [I also] invite them in[to] the classroom. We do a lot of that. . . . . That's really to get to know them.

- What are some ways you have benefited from getting to know your parent and caregiver community?

Katherine said, "I always reach out to parents" in order to learn more about students out of school. The parents' and caregivers' information fills in missing details of the picture Katherine creates about each student. For example, listening carefully to the parents' and caregivers' perspectives can help teachers understand student learning needs and observed classroom behavior. It affects how the teacher might consider approaching and supporting students in the classroom. Parents and caregivers can also play an important role in supporting student learning at home.

- What are some examples from your teaching experience when you found that getting to know a parent or caregiver informed your understanding of a student?

Rachel described how the building of relationships with parents and caregivers through the frequent sharing of information positively influences her teaching practice. To Rachel, the relationship can become a particularly rewarding point of positive connection when both teacher and parent or caregiver share a deep caring for the student:

Communicating with parents is extremely important . . . for the success of the kids . . . because if you don't communicate with [parents, you can miss out on important information]. Sometimes there is stress at home. . . . Talking with [parents] and finding out if there is stuff going on at home or if the kids need extra help with things, . . . [just] having that communication with parents is really important. . . .

It really is special when you can build relationships with these [students], and I think . . . when you talk to the parents, I think it means a lot to *them* when they know that you know their kid. I mean, [when] you have parents that say, "You *really* know [my child]. . . . That's exactly who they are." [That's special]. . . . I [also] think that [it] is important . . . for parents to know that their kids are safe and they're in a good environment and [that] you are going to do the best you can for them.

Katie shared how investing time in cultivating positive bonds with parents and caregivers makes her job of teaching over the course of the year much easier:

> Connecting with the families is huge. . . . When I first start working with the kids in September, I always connect with the parents. I call [about] good things. . . . If you get the parents to be a partner in . . . education, it makes your job so much easier. It's not like "us versus them." It should never be that. And, I think . . . [connecting with families] is just a huge part of [teaching success].

Later, Katie described how technology has supported her connections with parents and caregivers:

> I have . . . a remind app, where [parents and caregivers] can talk to me . . . privately via an app, and I can send out messages, like "Don't forget. . . . Book order money is due Friday," or whatever. . . . I have parents who contact me weekly on that. Or even just [a parent will contact me and say], "Oh, so and so forgot their homework, are you still there?" And I'll take a picture [of the homework] and send it, just because I check my phone a lot, and everything comes to the phone. So just . . . having the connection—even if it's a silly thing like that—[the parents] appreciate it.

- What boundaries, if any, do you establish with your students' parents and caregivers regarding your availability after school, in the evenings, and on weekends?
- What are some ways you manage your time and availability so you are able to be responsive to parents' and caregivers' needs while also setting aside time to renew and recharge yourself?

Like Barb, Katherine, Rachel, and Katie, Kim values the cultivation of positive and productive relationships with parents and caregivers. She tries to have parents and caregivers involved in a variety of ways and aims to establish clear lines of communication. For example, Kim said, "It is something I ask parents at curriculum night. . . . [I say], 'I don't want to know your personal business, but if there is a change [in your family situation], you need to let me know, because it does help me to understand [your child].' . . . It's invaluable to know those kinds of things."

That said, later Kim added how difficult it can be sometimes to forge a positive relationship with some students' family members:

> I do find it harder with some of the students' . . . parents with . . . addiction problems . . . [or if the parents are] coming out of, you know, bad relationship after bad relationship, that the children are seeing [and experiencing each day]. . . . I find that it's harder for me to [connect with and] understand where [those parents] are coming from. But, as a result, . . . I gravitate towards those kids. . . . I just try and do what I can [for those students]. [I] make those connections . . . [and build positive] relationships with those children.

- What do you do to establish and nurture a positive relationship with your students' parents and caregivers?
- Which aspects of your social and emotional skill set—self-awareness, self-management, social awareness, relationships skills, and responsible decision-making—tend to come into play when establishing and developing teacher–parent and teacher–caregiver relationships?[3]

PROACTIVELY SHARING THE POSITIVE

The educators not only celebrate successes with students in the classroom. Katie and others brought up how important it is to share those positives with the students' parents and caregivers, as well. Whether via brief exchanges at pick-up or drop-off; through quick phone calls, e-mails, and short notes sent home; or interactive apps, this communication highlighting the positives serves to enhance the teacher–parent or teacher–caregiver relationship. The information sometimes relates to academics, but the teachers also tell parents and caregivers positive stories of student effort, attitude, and kindness to others.

Suzy shared an example that had happened at pick-up at the end of a recent school day. It involved one of her current students who, in prior years, had a negative reputation and very difficult time at school. When Suzy looked out the window and saw that student's parent waiting outside for her son, she went "out and [told] his mom the little things that he did that [day that] helped another student." It was a really positive exchange and a celebration of who this mother's son was as a classmate.

- How might hearing positive information about their children influence parents and caregivers?

- How could it potentially affect the parent's or caregiver's interest in the school–home partnership over the course of the year and in future years?
- What has been your experience sharing positive information with parents and caregivers?

Suzy went on to say that throughout the day, she regularly seeks out and "really [tries] to find those good things that [the student] is doing" so she has even more good news to share with his mom.

- Consider what you have read in previous chapters about positive emotion and perception. How might intentionally seeking, finding, and sharing positive student information contribute to Suzy's experience of her work and the habits of noticing she develops?

HANDLING AN UPSET PARENT OR CAREGIVER

Fourth-grade teacher Katie is proud of the relationship she works hard to forge with her students' parents and caregivers, especially those considered "difficult" by others in the school. Listening carefully and acknowledging the parent's or caregiver's experiences, thoughts, and feelings is the core of her approach.

- Have you ever experienced a negative or upset parent or caregiver? If so, what approaches have you used that have influenced your success?

Katie gave an example of how she handles conversations with upset parents:

> I think . . . if you validate their feelings first and foremost, if they are aggravated about something, let them vent, and [then say something] like, "You know what. I can see you're frustrated. I completely understand why you're frustrated." . . . It kind of takes them down a notch because, if they feel like you are not listening to them, they're not going to stop with that feeling, and you're going to get nowhere. . . .
>
> [I] had one parent who was [still] *so frustrated* about something that happened [back] in kindergarten! [I was thinking], "We are in fourth grade, like, let's get beyond . . . kindergarten," [but I said to the parent], "I can see that frustrated you. I understand. That must have been a really stressful time."
>
> And then, I kind of gradually [got into the] year, and that parent was so much better! Like, such a nightmare in [the past] and [a] huge difference in fourth. . . . I don't know if it was just because I let her vent [during] that first

phone call, and [then I] said, "No, I completely understand why you were frustrated. That would have made me upset, too." . . .

[After that, I] just kind of [kept] in touch with her—[calling about] good things. . . . I mean, I've called and said, "Oh my gosh, I just wanted to share with you, so and so had such a *great* day today, and I wanted to let you know that they helped their friend out on the playground or whatever." Something [their child] did totally not related to anything . . . academic maybe but just that they were being a good person, and . . . the parent's like, "*Oh my god*, thank you so much for calling me!" Like, it made their whole day. So . . . taking the time to call. You know, . . . I think if the kids go home happy, and [the students] say they like school, that kind of helps, too, but . . . parent contact is huge, . . . especially with the difficult ones.

- What are some things that parents and caregivers do that might cause them to be identified as "difficult"? What might be some reasons parents and caregivers do what they do?
- In what ways might this reputation of "difficult parent" influence what each teacher sees, thinks, feels, and believes when meeting the parent for the first time? What connections, if any, can you make between this "difficult parent" label and your experiences with "Two Scenarios About Crossing a Room" in Part II and what you read about reputations in Chapter 2?

Chapter Nine

Relationships With Colleagues

The work of adults in schools is not an individual endeavor; each school community is characterized by interdependence. Researchers have found the quality of the adult relationships plays a significant role in school success.[1] As Bryk and Schneider state, "relationships are the lifeblood of activity in a school community. The patterns of exchanges . . . and the meanings that individuals draw from these interactions can have profound consequences on the operation of schools."[2]

In this chapter, you will hear how collegial relationships affect and inform the exemplary practitioners' experience of teaching as well as the quality of their practice. In order to make the shared information more meaningful, imagine you were asked to co-lead a new initiative in your educational setting with two colleagues:

- Who are the two people you would *want* in your group? Why?
- If those two people ended up in your group, how might your relationships with those colleagues influence the quality of your behavior, engagement, enthusiasm, and participation?
- Who are the two people you would *rather not* have in the group? Why?
- If those two people ended up in your group, how might your relationships with those colleagues influence the quality of your behavior, engagement, enthusiasm, and participation?

In each of these scenarios, how might the quality of the relationships influence the work that gets done, what doesn't get done, how it gets done, and why it gets done?

LISTENING, COMPASSION, AND SELF-COMPASSION

It is important to note that every exemplary teacher identified listening to colleagues as an important influence for successful teaching. In addition, nearly all teachers spoke effusively about at least one trusted colleague whose support was crucial to their educational outcomes. For example, Rachel said,

> I think it's . . . *really* those relationships—the communication—having a good team to work with. I think *that* is extremely important. To [be] able to bounce ideas off each other. [I] talk to my two [grade-level] colleagues all the time . . . because you know you can try things . . . a million different things, and [they] might not work, but the one thing the other teacher says could work perfectly, so that communication . . . is extremely important.

- How might knowing she has two colleagues to "bounce ideas off of" influence Rachel's experience of her work?

Rachel went on to say that teachers are "hard on themselves." That self-critical tendency coupled with the complex challenges and competing priorities that feature prominently in the teaching role can amplify the teacher's experience of the difficulties. According to Emma Seppala, science director of Stanford University's Center for Compassion and Altruism Research and Education, a wide base of research has found that "self-criticism destroys our resilience."[3] People who tend to beat themselves up have greater depression and anxiety, along with a reduced ability to bounce back and learn from mistakes.

In contrast, research suggests self-compassion reduces feelings of stress, lowers cortisol levels, lessens fear of failure, increases motivation to improve oneself, and enhances resilience. Seppala states,

> Self-compassion is the ability to be mindful of your emotions—aware of the emotions that are going on inside whenever you fail at something. It doesn't mean you identify with them; you can just observe and notice them, without feeding the fire. Self-compassion also involves understanding that everyone makes mistakes and that it's part of being human. And it is the ability to speak to yourself the way you would speak to a friend who just failed, warmly and kindly.[4]

In addition to developing self-compassion for oneself, Seppala offers cultivating compassion for others, nurturing positive connections with others, and practicing mindful breathing techniques as four research-based approaches that help calm the mind during stressful experiences.[5] To further explore this and related topics, please see the information listed under Mindfulness, Compassion, and Gratitude and also Faculty Protocols and Activities in appendix F.

Rachel is quick to emphasize how regularly communicating with her colleagues helps her unpack her understanding of challenging situations. Through those conversations, Rachel gains perspective and finds solutions. The kind, compassionate, mutual connection she experiences within her highly valued teacher-teacher relationships helps Rachel learn and grow. They are a source of energy. Rachel's comments suggested that each teacher's sense of capacity is enlarged by what they create in their interactions with one another. The positive relationships foster growth.

These ideas align with those put forth in the Relational-Cultural Theory (RCT) that centers on the role that connection, culture, and community plays in human experience. Each person's development does not occur in a vacuum.[6] It happens within a relational-cultural context: "Growth-fostering relationships are a central human necessity. Chronic disconnection, whether on an interpersonal or societal scale, is a primary source of human suffering."[7]

- What are some ways your relationships with colleagues influence your ability to negotiate hardship, learn, and grow?

Kim also spoke about how much she values her collegial relationships. She learns so much from listening carefully to her colleagues sharing of their successes and challenges. She always tries to learn from their experiences. She also relayed how important it is to ask for help from others when you need it:

> When listening to a colleague who is talking about . . . a [student] and how they've come so far and [how they have] turned [things] into a success, [I am always] taking [lessons] from my colleagues' experiences]. But [I] also [use] them as a resource when [I'm] having a problem, too, you know? You can't be too proud! (Laughs) . . . Seeking help when you need it and definitely having people you can vent to, that you know aren't judging you, [is so important, especially] when you're having one of those years.

- Kim mentioned venting, not judging, listening, and learning in her remarks. How do her comments fit with your experiences of sharing with colleagues?
- Who do you reach out to for support? How would you characterize your relationship with that person?

Katherine's colleagues, with whom she can openly share her lack of success and talk through her teaching challenges, reduce her feeling of isolation as a teacher. Her professional relationships, characterized by honesty and vulnerability, bolster Katherine's sense of efficacy as well as her energy level. She really appreciates collaborating with her caring and thoughtful colleagues. She knows they are there for her and they want to help her address challenging questions and concerns:

> Having [colleagues] who you can lean on and . . . talk to [is so important]. . . . I think you can't do it alone. It's definitely a collaborative profession. . . . When you [can] collaborate—when you [can] talk to a colleague and [say], "I don't know what's going on! This [student] is doing this, this, and this. What do you think?"
>
> I think it is really important [to] know you have [that kind of] a relationship with your colleagues [and that] you can . . . [talk with them] because you *can't* . . . know the answer for everything—you just *can't*. And then . . . also being open minded, too. Realizing that it might just not be *one reason* why that child is behaving that way.

- How might those positive professional relationships influence Katherine's daily approach to her work?
- How might knowing she has trusted colleagues whom she can talk to affect Katherine's perception of teaching difficulties right when they happen?

Rachel, Kim, and Katherine highlighted the importance of listening to colleagues. However, listening with openness to others is not always easy. Wanda shared that, in the past, she found that truly listening to some of her colleagues was quite challenging:

> I think [teacher-teacher] communication is very important—being able to listen to others—even if you don't agree with them. That was a lesson that I had to learn. There are people who have legitimate information to share. They may

be the boastful ones, but [it is important to] always take the time to listen because... I think we can all build our expertise on others' experiences.

- What helps you remain open and curious when colleagues offer ideas?
- What inhibits your ability to listen well to a colleague?

As mentioned elsewhere, teaching requires self-awareness, self-management, social awareness, relationship skills, and responsible decision-making, also known as the five core competencies of social and emotional learning.[8] Jillian spoke about how her relationship with a colleague in a nearby room supports her ability to bring the best of what she has to offer to her teaching. This is especially true when Jillian finds herself getting upset: "Sometimes I do need a minute.... I'll go [and ask] my colleague—[she] and I are very close—[and] sometimes she'll step in for a minute, ... just to give me a minute to regroup.... It's nice to have that support."

- How might knowing she has that level of collegial support influence Jillian's overall sense that she can handle upsetting experiences with equanimity?

Jillian and her colleague have set up an informal system to address the need to step outside the classroom for a moment to regroup. Some schools recognize how this type of teacher support is helpful for reducing staff stress levels. At Fall-Hamilton Elementary School in Nashville, Tennessee, the staff have a formal texting procedure called Tap-In/Tap-Out.[9] The staff schedule is organized so that there is always someone available to step in for another staff member. In this school, sometimes needing to ask for help is both expected and supported.

- What are some strategies you use when you need a minute to regroup?

TEACHER DEMORALIZATION, HOPELESSNESS, AND HOPE IN ACTION

Teaching is complex and challenging work. It requires intellectual, emotional, and interpersonal skill to negotiate the job's many competing priorities (e.g., content scope, teaching methodology, testing requirements, time constraints, differing student needs and interests). Educational processes emphasize individual student development, often via large- and small-group teaching methods, within a larger culture of public evaluation, judgment, and criticism.[10]

Education reform initiatives have taken a variety of approaches (e.g., national standards, school reorganizations, curriculum changes, curriculum content and pedagogy training, data collection, increased student testing). Notably, even when the improvement is widely viewed as necessary and well conceived, the nature of the change process itself can cause change fatigue and teacher dissatisfaction, affecting retention and stress.[11] Too many simultaneous improvement initiatives along with frequent shifting of priorities can negatively affect educator efficacy when too much is expected within too short a time.[12]

As referenced in Chapter 3, Bowdoin College's Doris Santoro identifies educator demoralization as an important influence in teacher turnover. Santoro explains,

> Demoralization is a form of professional dissatisfaction that occurs when teachers encounter consistent and pervasive challenges to enacting the values that motivate their work. Teachers who experience demoralization believe that the school practices or policy mandates that they are expected to follow are harmful to students or degrading to the profession and that their attempts to alter them have been fruitless.[13]

In a similar vein, during her exemplary teacher research interview, Patty brought up how hopeless some teachers feel. Speaking slowly and thoughtfully, Patty said, "[Some teachers] are tarnished a little bit by (pause) the job or worn down by (pause) years of . . . difficult situations where they feel their voice isn't heard or just tired of doing . . . differentiating instruction for kids, . . . [dealing] with [a difficult] family, . . . and that sort of thing, so I don't know. (pause) . . . There's a sense of hopelessness."

It is not surprising that researchers have found that hopelessness affects people's ability to apply the best of what they have to offer to their work.[14] Rego, a leading researcher studying workplace hope, describes how hope and intelligence reinforce each other to positively affect productivity and creativity.[15] When people feel hopeless at work, their intelligence remains an underutilized dormant resource.[16]

- How has hope and/or hopelessness influenced your ability to bring your best to your work?

Lopez suggests that hope in action involves three interrelated parts—meaningful goals, agency thinking, and pathway thinking—that act as a feedback loop for human behavior:

1. For the most hopeful people, a few well-considered *meaningful goals* provide direction and purpose for their actions. These people are clear about who they want to be and what they are moving toward.
2. *Agency thinking* relates to what people see as their individual strengths, skills, and attributes. It also is the awareness of various networks of people and other supports that can be marshaled to help fuel movement toward personally meaningful goals.
3. *Pathway thinking* involves consideration and analysis of multiple ways forward that lead to personally meaningful goals. It also includes the expectation and understanding that challenges lie on each path.

When one of the three parts weakens in some way, people experience a loss of hope.[17]

- Think of a time when you have experienced a loss or renewed sense of hope. Using Lopez's hope-in-action structure as a guide, what insight can you gain about your experience?

The exemplary teachers have relationships, priorities, and practices that nurture their sense of hope (personally meaningful goals, agency thinking, and pathway thinking) in an ongoing way. Hope affects the teachers' sense of capacity, energy, and tenacity. It also may provide insight into their ability to avoid burnout and cultivate success.

Hope serves as a motivational energy allowing for greater use of a person's abilities.[18] Interestingly, researchers have found that hope can act as a contagion; it can spread between people and among groups.[19] According to Lopez, a "hopeful student can achieve a letter grade higher than a less hopeful student of equal intellect."[20]

- What relationship have you found between hope and learning?
- When has hope served to spur you forward during a challenge?
- What are some ways you nurture hope in yourself and others?

To learn more about hope, please see appendix E.

Chapter 9

TEACHER CONVERSATIONS

Conversations between people are created and maintained by each person's individual decision-making about what, how, and when to contribute to the exchange.[21] Conversations have the potential to enliven as well as deflate. While nearly all the educators spoke positively about their colleagues' positive influence on their success, some also shared how the nature of other teacher conversations drain energy and squelch enthusiasm.

Suzy spoke about a powerful experience she had during her first year of teaching that involved a group of experienced and extremely negative teachers. Observing their teacher conversations significantly shaped the teacher Suzy has become:

> When I first started, there was an older group of teachers here, who were on their way out. [They were extremely negative.] . . . I started to almost resent the negativity—there was negative talk before school, negative talk after school, negative talk during lunch—about students. . . . As a new teacher [and] a young mom, I [began to] resent it. I wouldn't want somebody talking about my child that way. To this day, I *will not* sit and talk negatively about my students. So it's almost [as if] I decided, I am *not* going to do that. . . . I am going to do the opposite [instead]. . . .
>
> [Those negative teachers] made an impact on me. . . . I would hear them saying the same things over and over and over and over. And [I thought], "Guess what. [The student] is not going to stop [being who he is], . . . so you can either learn to appreciate it, or you can just continue to be driven crazy." (laughs) . . . [It] was a valuable learning experience for me back in those [early] days [as a teacher].

- How might negative teacher talk influence the speaker? How might negative teacher talk influence the listener?
- What might be some reasons teachers talk negatively?

Deborah described how new ideas are "not always welcomed" by some of her colleagues. She spoke about how she is always more than willing to "share what I do. I am willing to help—I'll do anything to help because I want [their students] to be as successful as my [students], . . . but not everybody wants things shared with them." Deborah went on to say,

> I'm not looking to shine. I'm not looking to generate attention. I'm not looking to give [colleagues] more work. . . . I think that we learn from one another as teachers. . . . I have a fabulous [grade-level] partner. . . . We do things together,

and we don't try to one-up one another. . . . I think that that's key in being successful, . . . taking it as a team approach. . . . When you try and one-up one another, . . . the kids lose [and] you lose. I think teaching is sharing.

- Consider the nature of teacher sharing in your setting. What variables do you think influence the quality of educator sharing where you work?

Wanda was the one teacher in the study who did not have an enthusiastic example of a positive relationship with a school colleague with whom she regularly collaborates. Instead, when speaking about colleagues, Wanda said,

> There are a number of people, [who I'll] say "Hi" to, and [then they respond with], "It's (heavy sigh) . . . it's only Tuesday." And I'll say to myself, "First of all, you woke up this morning, you have a loving husband, you have healthy children, you have a job, you have a new car, you have a place up north." . . .
>
> You know, it's like, people are not grateful for the . . . things in their lives, and I can't tell you how that will tick me off. It . . . it really, sets me off, so that I have to kind of, like regroup. [I say to myself,] "Okay, let it go. There is nothing you can do about it." But it's just . . . I wouldn't greet you like that! So it's kind of like a respect thing. . . . "If you need help, please! My door is open." But I cannot stand [their] negativity. I can't stand [the negative] attitude [of some of my colleagues].

- How do adults greet other adults in your school?
- What difference does that exchange make to you?

Positive collegial greetings are highlighted as a micropractice by the Collaborative for Academic, Social, and Emotional Learning to nurture development of a positive adult school community. Practices that signal engagement and appreciation, such as the use of attentive listening skills and verbal check-ins (e.g. "How are you?" "Look forward to seeing you later"), support development of productive adult relationships in schools.[22]

- What influence might adult-adult greetings have on the students who are watching the adults?

For further ideas, please see Faculty Protocols and Activities in appendix F.

Chapter 9

THE TEACHERS' ROOM

According to Case-Western Reserve Distinguished University Professor David Cooperrider, "we live in worlds our conversations create."[23] How would you describe the world that teacher conversations in your school create?

- What kinds of conversations do you hear in the teachers' room? What world is created in the teachers' room?
- How often do you go into the teachers' room?

Three of the exemplary teachers who taught in three different schools specifically highlighted their avoidance of the teachers' room as a positive influence on their success as teachers. Deborah described how she began eating in her classroom a number of years ago when she had an extremely difficult class. During that year, Deborah "just needed a little quiet" before the challenging group of students returned from recess.

Deborah said, in her teachers' room, "You can't help but hear . . . 'Oh, wait till you get this one!' [or] 'Oh, the class I have this year!'" Deborah found eating in her classroom so helpful to her well-being that she continues to do it today. But now, a few colleagues join her, and they enjoy chatting over lunch together. Deborah views her collegial relationships with these colleagues as central to her work and success.

Wanda also spoke about avoiding her teachers' room but for a different reason. Wanda finds the teachers' room conversations dominated by boasters who show off, saying, "Well, I did this, and I know that" throughout lunch. To Wanda, this kind of sharing is not helpful to others.

- Wanda used the term *boaster* in her comments. Have you ever heard a teacher boast? If so, what does that look like and sound like?
- What is the difference between boasting and sharing successes?
- In what ways can the quality of the teacher-teacher relationship affect the perception and interpretation of teacher behavior as boasting?

Although Barb highly values her relationships with colleagues, she has intentionally avoided the teachers' room throughout her long career. She wants to guard herself from hearing the negative information shared there. Barb said, if she does hear her colleagues' negative commentary about a student or students' family members,

I have to kind of take a deep breath and step back, and I almost try to erase what I heard, and I start from that point on. . . . [I don't] want to hear [it] because negativity and preconceived ideas slow you down and hold you back and don't let you see the whole picture of a [student].

[What those teachers are talking about] could be one moment in time. It could have been one situation. It could have been the dynamics of the classroom. I don't know. I wasn't there. So what I don't know I put on the back burner because I don't know all the other dynamics that . . . happened in that particular situation.

Instead of spending time in the teachers' room, Barb works hard to forge positive relationships with colleagues in settings that are more formally structured, such as in professional development workshops or staff meetings. She said, "I think finding positive ways to interact with your colleagues in a professional manner helps you to be successful."

- How do you interact with your colleagues?
- In what ways can the teachers' room discussions affect the reputations of students or their parents and caregivers?
- If you could create an ideal teachers' room, what would it be like?

SEEING THINGS DIFFERENTLY AND SEEING DIFFERENT THINGS

Humans cannot see everything that is right in front of them. The human perception system is just too limited.[24] Barb spoke about the value of having access to different people's perspectives. She finds it helpful to have another set of eyes in the classroom. To Barb, hearing about what her aide notices and how she interprets situations gives her an advantage as a teacher. Sometimes Barb and her aide notice the same things. Sometimes their interpretations of the same things differ. Sometimes different things stand out in a situation, so they see different things.

- Have you ever been in someone else's classroom and seen something that the teacher missed?
- Have you ever had someone in your room share something that you missed?
- Have you ever had an interpretation of a situation that differed from others who observed the same situation?

It was clear from her comments that Barb wants to learn about what other adults in her classroom notice and how they interpret what they have seen. She values different perspectives, whether from her aide, with whom she regularly shares, or other people who observe her teaching in the classroom. Barb gave an example of one way sharing with her aide expands understanding:

> I look at . . . the whole sometimes, the whole picture. Where sometimes, others look at specific details within that picture. . . . It's how [we each] perceive things that are happening. . . . It's hard to really explain, but [we see different things. It] does happen—often. What we do in [my] classroom is we share those, and . . . we learn from each other. . . . We're blessed to be able . . . to do that. Not all classrooms run that way. . . . It helps me then tune into and rethink how to look at something. . . . For me, [it] helps.
>
> [My aide may be noticing] my working with [a] particular [student or] observing a particular technique I used that I thought really worked well. . . . [But] then, when reflecting [together] or [listening to] someone else's point of view, [it leads to my] realizing it may not have worked as well as I thought it did.

Through sharing with one another, they both become more aware of what they each may have missed. Their open and honest relationship and frequent communication provides Barb with greater insight into what is happening in her classroom and why it might be happening. After they explore their different perspectives and diverse opinions, they each end up seeing and understanding more of what happens in the classroom. To further explore some of the variables that influence why we see things the way we do, please see appendix D.

- What might be some ways that this teacher-aide relationship influences Barb's teaching success? What qualities or characteristics are needed by each person to have this kind of professional relationship?
- Think about times when you shared your perspective with other people who saw different things or saw things differently than you. What can be challenging about those conversations?
- What are some short-term and long-term consequences (intended or unintended) when diverse views are squelched?

June also shared an example of a time when she turned to a colleague to gain a different perspective. In June's situation, she and her colleague saw the same student behavior, but they interpreted the student's behavior differently. June began by describing how the student was "like nails on chalkboard. . . . . She drove me nuts. . . . It was getting to the point where, the minute I'd see [the student in the hall], my blood pressure would go up. Every morning. Like ugh!" This troubling self-awareness led June to reach out to a colleague who also taught the student. June asked her colleague, "How do you handle her?"

To her great surprise, June found that her colleague enjoyed the student tremendously. Her colleague found the student funny. While the student exhibited similar behavior in both educational settings, the other teacher did not interpret the behavior or the student with annoyance; instead, she saw the humor in it.

Learning more about the way her colleague perceived the student's behavior and hearing how her colleague spoke about the student was helpful to June. It really made June think more about what she was "looking at. . . . [It made me realize] there is something about that [student] that is funny. And it kind of made me step back." June realized she was not seeing all there was to see in that student. June also began to think about how she could interpret the student's behavior differently. June asked herself, How was it that "what I found annoying, [her colleague] found . . . comical?"

Hearing her colleague's very different perception of the student shifted the content of June's automatic internal storyline that began when June saw the student walking down the hall. June intentionally sought to add to and alter the clear picture she had created about that student. With applied focus, curiosity, and openness, June worked hard to change how she perceived the student.

June said, when she thought more about her colleague's approach to and view of the student, "it made [the student's behavior] more tolerable. . . . I tried to find the humor in it. . . . And I kind of did." By asking for help from a colleague and learning additional ways to view and understand the student's behavior, June augmented how she saw and interpreted the student's natural way of being. As a result, June's experience with the student shifted.

In this example, June used self-awareness and applied intrapersonal curiosity to understand her automatic negative reaction to her student. Her solid and trusting relationship with a colleague made it possible for her to honestly share an increasing dislike of a student.

- What might have happened if June had not sought a different perspective about the student?
- Have you ever had a student who pushed your buttons? If so, what are some ways you managed that situation successfully?
- What influences the internal storyline you create about each of your students?

According to Harvard University's Susan David, the "way we navigate our inner world—our everyday thoughts, emotions, and self-stories—is the single most important determinant of our life success. It drives our actions, careers, relationships, happiness, health; everything."[25]

THE JOY OF SHARING WITH OTHERS

All but one of the exemplary teachers in the study had at least one person with whom they shared regularly. Some teachers had their collegial conversations every day while driving to school; others popped into their colleague's room at some point before each school day began. Some teachers met in their classrooms during lunch or free blocks, or they touched base after school. All who spoke about their positive collegial relationships deeply appreciate their connections with fellow teachers. For example, Patty said, "I love sharing with people, and I'm always, you know, handing out things that I found or whatever, and so I think if you do that, hopefully people will give back . . . and make it a two-way street."

Rachel highlighted how important it was to be able to savor what is working well with her colleagues:

> Sharing those successes! I think being able to share them with my colleagues and being able to say, "Oh, so and so did this!" It just makes you feel better. . . . I think sharing it is really helpful because you can tell yourself all the time, "I did great!" (Laughs) "What a good job!" or give yourself a pat on the back, but I don't think it means as much as if other people are saying it [with you], too.

The kind of collegial celebration of successes described by Rachel can nourish and spread positive emotion. According to Lambert and colleagues, "if the receiver of the good news actively and constructively responds, it can often provide a boost in wellbeing to both people involved in the conversation."[26] This finding concerning active constructive responding may provide insight into the way their positive collegial relationships serve as another source of energy for the exemplary teachers.

The opposite of acting like a killjoy, a person who uses active constructive responses instead explores and promotes the savoring of the good news. Nonverbally they respond in ways that connote caring and interest. The teller of the good news has an opportunity to expand on, relive parts of, and more greatly appreciate different aspects of that which went well.[27] To learn more, please see the information listed under Faculty Protocols and Activities in appendix F.

Celebrating successes through sharing positive stories can also nurture a sense of hope. For example, as Kim highlighted with collegial sharing, colleagues may learn specific techniques and approaches to enhance their teaching practices. It is important to note that the positive storytelling has inherent value, even if no specific pedagogical learning occurs. In *Hope in the Age of Anxiety*, Scioli and Biller explain that, throughout human history, the sharing of stories, myths, folktales, fables, and the like have cultivated hope in the listeners.[28]

- Think of some stories that you find inspirational. What's your hunch about how hearing stories cultivates hope?
- In what ways do your positive collegial relationships influence your energy level and experience of hope?

Katie's positive collegial relationships play a significant role in her success. She spoke about helping and enjoying one another:

> I think, just being in a good place [with each other], where you feel like [you can ask for help and support]. I can [say to a colleague], "Hey do you have anything for this [topic]?" And they say [with enthusiasm], "Oh yes, yes, yes!" . . . [Sharing] makes your job so much easier than planning alone. . . . [The] interaction [with newer teachers is helpful, too]. . . . They can remind you [about what you did in the past]. "Oh gosh, I remember I did that 10 years ago. I forgot about doing that!"

Katie's close relationships with her colleagues influence her experience of her daily work and overall sense of capacity. Bryk and Schneider describe how "important consequences play out in the day-to-day social exchanges within a school community. . . . Good schools depend heavily on cooperative endeavors. Relational trust is the connective tissue that binds individuals together to advance the education and welfare of students."[29]

Bryk and Schneider researched the Chicago Public School System and identified relational trust in the adult school community as a strong predictor of school improvement success.[30] It also affects teacher burnout.[31] This topic is further explored in the next chapter.

Kayla's sentiments capture the zest common in the exemplary teachers' comments about their positive relationships with colleagues. Kayla said one of her "greatest joys as a teacher is working with other teachers and creating lessons together and seeing how other teachers teach. It's important not to teach in a vacuum. You have to be able to say, 'Oh, . . . I love how she introduced that lesson. I never would have done it that way!' or 'Gee, I had this great idea!' and share it." Kayla's comments relate to Cooperrider's description of the power of appreciation:

> Relationships come alive where there is an appreciative eye, when we take the time to see the true, the good, the better, and the possible in each other and our universe of strengths, and when we use this concentrated capacity to activate conversations that open our world to new possibilities, elevate collective genius and purpose, and build bonds of mutual regard and positive power—not "power over" but "power to."[32]

- How do your relationships with colleagues positively affect your "power to"?
- What do you think are the prerequisites for positive and productive collegial conversations?

Chapter Ten

The Administration of Schools

In this chapter, the exemplary teachers share administration practices that support and inhibit their work. To start this exploration, identify what you believe are the markers of good school administration.

- What does it take to be a helpful and effective school administrator?
- In what ways do administrators influence how learning happens in your educational setting?

In *A Practice Agenda in Support for How Learning Happens*, Berger, Berman, Garcia, and Deasy state,

> Research has made clear that social, emotional, and cognitive skills work in concert to build students' success in school and in life. . . . The meaningful and effective cultivation of each student's social, emotional, and cognitive development does not come from purchasing a program or mandating a new policy.
>
> [Instead] it comes from districts, schools, organizations, and communities working together to forge a vision for students' comprehensive development; from building respectful learning communities that value all students and staff and foster positive relationships; from teaching social, emotional, and cognitive skills explicitly and embedding them into all academic instruction; from prioritizing and building adult capacity to model and teach these skills; and from working across schools and community organizations to align and collaborate for the good of all children.[1]

- In what ways do these research ideas align with your school's vision and practices?

POLICIES, PAPERWORK, AND POLITICS

The exemplary teachers spoke about how school administrators make decisions that directly affect important teaching and learning variables. Jillian, Katherine, Barb, Debbie, and Patty identified how some of their administration's policies, required paperwork, and politics impede their ability to do their job well. Jillian's comments capture the frustration arising from being required to attend to the details of yet another unexpected and influential mandate created by others working outside the classroom:

> All these new policies and standards is just overload sometimes. . . . I am trying to better myself and go to school, as well, so . . . on top of outside personal obligations and school, . . . it's a lot. . . . Having those extra mandates come down and having those extra protocols that we have to do, it's stressful. . . . Those [are] negative things, . . . when you come in and you're like, "Uh, what's going to be new? What is going to be thrown upon us today?" . . . So that can get frustrating.

- What do you make of Jillian's phrase "thrown upon us"? How does that sentiment fit or not fit with your experience?

Katherine described her current school administration's emphasis on data collection. While Katherine agrees that data can be useful, how it is gathered and used seems unhelpful:

> Not to be cliché, but it really is [important to take] into consideration the whole child. I think [we can] get so wrapped up nowadays in . . . [the] administrative stuff that is so unimportant, that I think you lose the sense of why we're here. . . . [We're] here to teach the children. A lot of administrators don't understand that. They just want to see data and data and data and data. . . . I think that [it is important to value] understanding the child, the *whole* child.

Barb also spoke about the "administrative stuff" that Katherine referenced. In particular, Barb described the level of additional paperwork that is now required as a regular part of her job. She said, when "you do one form for one person [and then you have to] do another form for another person. That takes away from me being productive."

- What helps you negotiate the policies and paperwork of teaching?

Debbie spoke about how hard it can be sometimes when the top school administrators in her town do not support the work of teachers. However, she has had to become savvy about how and when to share her frustrations. Debbie relayed how knowing the politics in the building and the town are also important to teaching success:

> Knowing who I can vent to and knowing who I can't vent to. . . . Sometimes you learn that in a bad way, and sometimes you learn it in a good way. . . . I know that there are people here who have my back no matter what (taps table). Sometimes I don't feel the top [town] administration has my back, but (pause) I know that there [are people here who do], and . . . I would move mountains for them.

Patty, who teaches in a different town, also spoke about how town and school politics encroach into and infiltrate the building. She explained how politics are especially influential during contract time:

> The politics that can go on in the town, budget-wise . . . [and in] the building, [can be difficult]. [Some] years are more negative than others, with things that don't even apply to me personally, but I can see that people are unhappy and . . . angry. . . . There's a lot of . . . [staff] conversations [and] negativity. . . . I think that that drags [all of us] down.
>
> That's not . . . a healthy, creative environment that you really came into this profession to be around. . . . I think that it can be very toxic. Even though you can't help but have an opinion about what's going on outside [your] own classroom, it . . . does drag you down over time.

Patty explained that, during the highly charged budget-allocation periods, conversations by town financial decision makers sometimes are divisive. Patty feels people who do not work in schools can oversimplify and undervalue the complexity of teaching. They also underestimate its importance: "You know, sometimes I feel like . . . people don't really understand what a good teacher does. . . . I don't know how to make that better. I am not a politician. But the news *has* to get out there. And . . . we [as colleagues] talk about [that]."

Patty also spoke about how teachers feel their goodwill and dedication is often taken for granted, and that that can leave lingering bitterness long after the contract has been signed:

> [During] contract time . . . things are *so* difficult. . . . [*Our* lives are affected. But] the teachers [will] always make it work. We will never let our [students]

go without. . . . [We] do what we have to do. . . . So as far as [the students] are concerned, they don't skip a beat. And as far as the parents go, they don't skip a beat because their day has not changed one iota. But I think, over time, [teachers] can get bitter about the fact that [what we do is] not recognized [or appreciated]. . . .

[People outside education don't value] what you need [to do] in order to make this work on a day-to-day basis. I think that that can drag you down. [But] I think if there's too many [teacher-teacher] conversations happening about how . . . awful it [all] is, that's just very disheartening.

- What do teachers tend to talk about in your school?
- Given the typical conversations that occur among adults, how easy or hard is it to be upbeat in your setting?

SOCIAL BONDS, RELATIONAL TRUST, AND EMOTIONAL CONTAGION

As mentioned in Chapter 3, Kayla experienced significant difficulties in the past when she was required by her previous school administration to use teaching materials that did not align with her students' learning needs. Later in the interview, Kayla spoke about how much she now appreciates the professional freedom granted by her current school leadership:

We are *very* lucky in this building that we have administration that supports us. . . . We are a Title I school, so we have funds that we can put into . . . supplemental things. We have a principal and an assistant principal that have said, "The frameworks are your curriculum. Everything else is a resource. You need to teach your curriculum." The [provided subject matter programs are now considered] a resource. Now . . . I can use *pieces* of the math program, but I can also go on and find other things that I think fit the developmental needs of my [students].

Kayla and her colleagues appreciate the trust and respect demonstrated by their principal and assistant principal. The positive administration-teacher relationship makes a difference. Positive relationships are crucial for the well-being of both students and adults in schools.

According to University of California, Santa Barbara, researchers Gable and Bromberg, the creation and maintenance of positive social bonds supports physical and mental health: "Processes such as the reduction of negative emotion, shaping the self-concept, support for personal goals, and eliciting positive emotions are [some examples of the] mechanisms through which [positive social bonds] have the potential to enhance well-being."[2]

- In what ways do the positive social bonds in your school community influence your work experience, energy level, and sense of well-being?

Katie, who does not teach in the same school as Kayla, also spoke about how important her principal's support is to her teaching success. Katie explained that some of her students have extremely difficult lives and, as a result, sometimes need extra support. Her principal has created systems and processes so teachers can make a quick call to the office to get their students what they need.

Her principal has also cultivated a positive adult school community. Katie knows her colleagues and trusts that they will support her students when they need extra help. She spoke about her school staffs' expertise, availability, and kindness:

> They are *very, very* kind and supportive and helpful if I have a student who's struggling. I can call and say, "Listen, so-and-so is having a really tough day. Would you mind if I sent him down?" [They say], "No, no, send him down." And they'll help. . . . It's not like you're alone. I mean, you can choose to be alone if you'd like, but (laughs), I prefer to [be able to say], "Hey, can you help me out here because he's really having a hard day?" It is *big*. You don't see that everywhere.

It was evident through this and Katie's other descriptions of her collegial relationships that her school community seems to have the four the markers of relational trust:

1. *Integrity*—Colleagues are committed to the welfare and education of students and "can be trusted to keep their word."[3]
2. *Competency*—Colleagues believe in each other's competency: "Colleagues have the knowledge, skill, and/or technical capacity to deliver on their intentions and promises."[4]
3. *Personal regard*—Colleagues are willing "to extend themselves beyond what is formally required . . . 'going the extra mile' for another person."[5]
4. *Respect*—In conversations throughout the school community, colleagues genuinely listen "to what each person has to say," and these views are taken "into account in subsequent actions. Even when peo-

ple disagree, individuals . . . still feel valued [because] others respect their opinions."[6]

Relational trust is also referenced in Chapter 9 as a foundational school success variable. While it is not the only factor required for school improvement, Bryk and Schneider found "evidence directly linking the development of relational trust in a school community and long-term improvements in academic productivity."[7] Without relational trust, sustained school improvement is less likely.[8]

- In what ways is relational trust nurtured in your school community?

June, who teaches in a different school from Kayla and Katie, described a time when she had a difficult relationship with a colleague. She expressed that she was glad that the teacher is no longer teaching at her school. The educator's contributions to grade-level collegial conversations were *not* helpful. She did not listen to others with attention and openness, and she did not have the students' best interests at heart. June said,

> [She] could not tolerate the kids who needed the extra help, the [students] who were needy. . . . She just had a hard time with those [students]. . . . Everyone here has a great heart, and we always talked about [her lack of tolerance]. . . . She would say the kids were "lazy" or the "apple doesn't far fall from the tree." She just couldn't have tolerance for them. . . . *No* other teacher [is] like that [here]. . . .
>
> [This school] is like a safe haven. It's a small school. Everyone knows each other. We know the needy kids. And if I need to help, I'll go! . . . I think that's the beautiful thing . . . of having a smaller school rather than those big complexes. We know who the [students] are that need the extra help . . . and the extra attention, . . . [and we give it]!

Suzy spoke of the impact of a current colleague who is consistently negative, arrives late, and leaves early. The teacher's reasons for the late arrivals and early departures have been found to be untruthful. The teacher exhibits a lack of integrity, and her treatment of students reflects a lack of competence. After describing the situation, Suzy said,

> [So] now, I have to cover her class again. It draws on you. It's draining emotionally. . . . I have never had a difficult working relationship with anyone in this school, so this [situation] is (pause), it's draining. . . . [That teacher] can't bring that . . . bad attitude into [this school]. . . . Just hearing [her]

yelling. (pause) . . . The screaming and the negativity—it's so draining on my soul, it really is, (pause) and then I worry about her [students].

Suzy went on to say in a relieved tone, "Fortunately . . . the administration is very well aware of it and hopefully will make some adjustments."

Having an administrator clearly attend to adult behavior that erodes relational trust is crucial to a high-functioning learning environment. Cranston highlights how "relational trust has to be built and sustained, and it has to be active. Principals need to work continually [on] the social network of the school. . . . this takes time, commitment, and effective communication."[9]

- In what ways can the actions of administrators positively or negatively influence the level of relational trust in schools?

Berger and colleagues offer administrators two related recommendations in *A Practice Agenda in Support of How Learning Happens*:

> Provide and prioritize ongoing professional learning opportunities for educators to support their own social and emotional skills and their ability to lead students' comprehensive growth. This professional learning has multiple benefits: it guides faculty in how to model and teach these skills; it strengthens the capacity and resilience of teachers; and it fosters a positive school culture.
>
> Support and hold all educators accountable for modeling social and emotional skills, holding this as central to faculty expectations, as a focus for school walkthroughs and for educator reflection and critique.[10]

Suzy echoed: "We all have lives outside of here, and they are not always roses and butterflies and sunshine, but we *cannot* bring that into the building."

As mentioned in earlier chapters, Wanda also finds some of her colleagues' pervasive negativity difficult to be around. She shared how it affects the collegial atmosphere and the students' experience of school: "The naysayers, the negative people really put a damper on things. . . . [And] those children have to sit in those [negative teachers'] rooms all day long. [Students] *feel* that because they are very sensitive to that—they *feel* that. They pick it up."

Becker, Goetz, Morger, and Ranellucci's research supports Wanda's assertions. They found the teachers' emotional messages affect their instructional message. Emotional contagion, an unintentional mimicry that occurs through mirror neurons, likely plays a role in these research outcomes.[11]

Mirror neurons are "brain cells that become active when an organism is watching an expression or behavior that they themselves can perform."[12]

Researchers in neuroscience, social psychology, communication research, and industrial-organizational psychology have all found evidence of human emotional contagion. Humans have the capacity to "catch" different people's emotions. For example, when listening to a person tell a sad story, the listeners may find themselves feeling more sadness as well without putting forth any intentional effort to do so.[13] Conversely, seeing people laugh or hearing a high-quality laugh track can influence a humor response in comedy viewers. University of Chicago professor of neurology and psychology Steven Small states, "When you smile or when you see someone smiling, the same regions of the brain are active. . . . If you see two people laughing at a joke you didn't hear, you may laugh anyway. There's a real imitative aspect of it. That's been demonstrated. There are overlapping areas [in the brain] for laughing and seeing laughter."[14]

- With the information about emotional contagion in mind, what emotion tends to spread between and among educators in your setting?

SEEING AND SHARING POSITIVES

Humans tend to view the negative and problematic features of a situation as more important than the positive that also exists in the same moment in time.[15] The negative in situations stands out. It captures and focuses attention. This normal human tendency, called negativity bias (introduced in Chapter 6), has helped humans survive as a species.

When time, attention, or resources are limited, the identification and fixing of what is wrong can seem like the highest priority. While tending to the negative is certainly important, seeing only the negative in a situation means seeing an incomplete picture of what is happening. Ignoring the value of what is working well is a missed opportunity. That said, when the immediacy of a negative experience is upon us, it can sometimes be hard to bring any worthwhile positives to mind. They just do not seem as relevant.[16]

This negative focus is consistent with much of Patty's experience in her school until very recently. Patty happily shared that, in the prior week, two outside curriculum experts observed one of her lessons. She received detailed feedback about her teaching. Patty said,

Afterwards . . . they said, "That was wonderful. . . . I wish I had a video camera." . . . And, you know, I felt like a little kid because [it] made me feel so good that someone was validating something that I do . . . because, I mean, . . . who is going to tell you that they think your lesson is great? . . . It just doesn't happen. . . .

It's just nice to know that what you are doing is okay, it's working, [and] someone is saying, "That looks great." . . . I think that it's nice to hear that once in a while. . . . It is nice to have people recognize what is done. . . . I think . . . [here] everybody is in their own little world. . . . [Opportunities to watch each other teach and opportunities for] collaboration are few and far between. . . .

I think people are always concerned about someone showboating or getting too much praise or [thinking] maybe "They're doing a better job than me" or whatever.

In contrast to Patty's school atmosphere, Jillian shared how helpful it is to have positive collegial relationships with her principal and colleagues. They point out her successes and highlight how her efforts help others. Jillian said,

> We have a strong support system here. . . . Getting that positive reinforcement from colleagues and from administration—that *really* makes a difference. Even just a small thank you. . . . You don't need a pat on the back, but sometimes it *is* nice to hear. Just with all those negative things coming down [on teachers] . . . [it is nice to hear] that you are doing something right.

Rachel, who teaches at a different school from Jillian, similarly shared how important her principal was to her success:

> My principal is . . . really good about telling us the positive things that she sees that we're doing [and also] . . . giving us pats on the back for little things, . . . and I think that makes a huge difference. Especially if you are ever feeling down, or you know, you have [a day] where you're like, "Oh (sigh), . . . that was a terrible lesson," like, "I didn't get anywhere"—but then, if [the principal] says something to you like, "Hey, by the way, I saw that so and so made progress, and it was only one point, but they made one point!" . . . Just those small, . . . recognizing those small successes, I think, gives you hope again.

- How does the principal noticing and highlighting small teacher successes align with the teachers noticing and highlighting small student successes?
- While it is important to focus on, understand, and address problems, just working on getting rid of problems does not automatically equate to thriving. What are some things that help you thrive?

PRODUCTIVE TEACHER SHARING

The role of teacher is complex. A number of the exemplary teachers emphasized the benefits of having more opportunities to share ideas in productive and positive ways with colleagues. Deborah emphasized the importance of teacher-teacher sharing to facilitate and enhance educational decision-making. In particular, Deborah suggested principals set aside more time for teacher-teacher discussion about the data collected:

> Why the heck are we collecting all this data if we're not going to talk about it? The reading teacher, the special ed teacher, [and] the aides . . . [all] come in [and work with my students periodically]. . . . I've got *all* this information that's sitting here (points to the pile of paper on her desk). But if [different people are] working with [my students] and . . . [they] don't know what this [data] is telling [us about those students, then why collect it?]
>
> So I think communication is huge. It can be as quick as [me asking the reading teacher], "Hey, what are you doing for [him during your lesson today?]" to [me saying], "I am trying [this technique] this week. What do you think? Can you carry it over into your times with him, too?"

- What are some ways important information is effectively communicated in your school?

In addition to sharing data and techniques, June explained how observing other educators in their classrooms potentially expands teacher beliefs about what is possible to achieve. For example, if colleagues who teach the same grade level are given the opportunity to watch each other teach, it might influence the observer's understanding of student capacities for that grade. June said, "I think [having] a lot more time for teachers to work with other teachers is huge because I think when you are in your own little room, you get too routine. . . . If you [get to talk together and also] go into other teacher's classes, [you see different things]. [You can leave thinking], 'Oh my god, if they can do this, I can do this!'"

June relayed a pivotal experience from very early in her career, when she got to observe a colleague teach a new form of journal writing: "[Her] kids wrote *three pages*. My kids [were writing] *three sentences*! *Oh my god*, I can expect more of them! . . . I came back [and made a few changes], and *boom* my kids were writing. That's *all* it took—[just watching her teach]. I'll *never* forget that moment!"

Often, the teachers in her building discuss how helpful watching each other and sharing together more would be, but June said, the administration are "so afraid to do that.... [They think] that we are going to waste time." According to DuFour, without the necessary information and support, teachers may end up wasting time. DuFour describes how just putting "teachers together in a room" and telling "them to collaborate" is not helpful. To DuFour, two conditions foster productive teacher-teacher collaborations: "first, absolute clarity about what [they're] collaborating on—what is the nature of the work, what is the right work—and second, [the provision of] supports so people can succeed at what they're being asked to do. If [administrators] fulfill those two things, collaboration will have a much greater impact."[17]

Patty also spoke about the importance of administrator support and clarity to facilitate productive teacher-teacher sharing. While Patty appreciates how her school administration has built in common planning blocks across grade levels so teachers can talk together, she wonders if the time could be better spent. She offered the suggestion that principals nurture a school culture where all teachers freely share what works. Patty described their current set-up:

> We [do] have our common planning time once a week as a team, ... and they meet here in my room.... We don't have an agenda from week to week. We discuss whatever is the most poignant or things that are coming up in our schedules or whatever.... It's a nice opportunity for us to just kind of make sure we are all on the same page....
>
> If it were up to me, I would take it a step further.... I would make it so that everyone brings something to the table, literally bring something to share, you know? ... Something that you feel like we all could benefit from.... It doesn't have to be anything fancy or take any extra time but maybe something that you've noticed that works or whatever.... I would love to see that, and I think that there are a lot of people that would like something like that....
>
> But I think [you need to] ... establish a rapport with people [first].... I think if [we] can establish the fact that no one is going to be judged and that you're ... here to give me something and I am here to give you something and ... [we all are] sharing in a nonthreatening way without ... people overseeing it, [it could work well].... [I'm talking about] creating an environment where people are comfortable and people have the time to sit [together and learn from one another].

- What have you found supports a productive use of teacher meeting time?

Sarah Fiarman, author of *Becoming a School Principal: Learning to Lead, Leading to Learn*, agrees with DuFour's assertions and Patty's remarks about teachers' use of precious common planning time[18]:

> Research has shown that teachers learn new practices through collaborating with peers. For this reason, [when I was a principal], I prioritized scheduling common planning time for teams at my school to meet each week. Over time, I learned that simply forming teams and scheduling time doesn't lead to improvement, however.
>
> While some teacher teams are able to pursue learning on their own, most need more explicit support to ensure meetings are productive and useful. Thus, at my school, grade-level team leaders learned protocols for identifying root cause, designing an inquiry cycle, soliciting critical feedback from teammates, and—importantly—they learned strategies for protecting an agenda's focus on practice rather than completing paperwork and other housekeeping.
>
> We used these strategies when the whole staff was together as well. One teacher noted that instead of staff meetings, we now had workshops where teachers worked together to examine instruction.[19]

For links to meeting materials referenced by Fiarman, please see Faculty Protocols and Activities in appendix F.

- Do you use protocols in your teacher–teacher and staff meetings to support productive conversation? If so, what influence has it made?

Interestingly, productive teacher-teacher collaboration is one of Santoro's suggestions for "remoralizing" demoralized teachers. As introduced in Chapter 3, there is a difference between teacher demoralization and burnout. According to Santoro, principals who understand the difference will be better able to support teachers effectively.[20]

For those educators who are becoming burned out, one beneficial principal support may relate to time management. For example, it may be helpful for principals to provide clear direction such that teachers can better negotiate the competing priorities they face so their time is managed effectively. Santoro identifies educator "self-care, mindfulness, and boundary setting" as some other recommendations.[21]

Demoralized teachers' needs are different. Santoro explains that they "need to gain more control over their profession, engaging in conversations with peers and bosses, to start to change what their job looks like."[22] Santoro shares that, during her 10 years of teacher research, she has seen educators "remoralized" in a variety of ways:

> It could be as simple as having a principal listen seriously to their concerns, even if big changes can't be made. It can be from engaging in activism, as teachers throughout the country have done [recently]. . . .
>
> Teachers can also reengage with their profession if they find an authentic professional community, even if that means connecting with local professors and taking on more work. While the immediate remedy for stressed teachers would seem to be having them do less, . . . sometimes it is about doing more.[23]

Although this book's emphasis relates to teacher turnover, it is important to note that administrator turnover is also a significant educational issue in the United States: "Nearly half of new principals leave their schools after three years, and nearly 20 percent leave every year."[24] Although the exemplary teachers did not specifically mention the frequency of administrative turnover, it is a variable influencing U.S. teachers' experience.

- What are some ways a change of leadership every one to three years can influence teaching and learning in a school?

COLLECTIVE EFFICACY

Since Stanford University's Albert Bandura's research was first completed in the 1970s, researchers across many domains have confirmed that, "when a team of individuals share the belief that through their unified efforts they can overcome challenges and produce intended results, groups *are* more effective."[25] According to John Hattie, laureate professor at the University of Melbourne, collective efficacy is a significant factor that influences student achievement.[26] Donohoo, Hattie, and Eells highlight how

> team members' confidence in each other's abilities and their belief in the impact of the team's work are key elements that set successful school teams apart. [However,] publicly seeking evidence of positive effects on student learning does not happen serendipitously or by accident and neither does a sense of psychological safety. School leaders must work to build a culture designed to increase collective teacher efficacy, which will affect teachers' behavior and student beliefs. . . . When teams of educators believe they have the ability to make a difference, exciting things can happen in a school.[27]

Collective educator efficacy is evident in June's remarks concerning the functioning of her current school. This is in sharp contrast to June's experience in her previous school district, which was so "dysfunctional" that she had to leave (see Chapter 3). Although changing school districts meant June lost her seniority and she took a financial hit, the benefits to her well-being were well worth it. June appreciates being a member of her current school community. Together, they are able to make substantive change in their students' lives. June spoke about how in her school there are students "who don't have it so good [in their lives]. And I know that, when they come in here, they feel loved. . . . I know that . . . I don't make a ton of money, but . . . I know that—at the end of the day—we are making a difference. We *totally* are. And I *know* that."

- What role does collective efficacy play in your school community?

III

Personal Practices and Skills

In the book *On Looking: A Walker's Guide to the Art of Observation*, Alexandra Horowitz shares her record of 11 walks "with expert seers" around a city block.[1] Each chapter contains the story of what one expert pointed out during their stroll together. Her walking companions included a geologist, a typographer, an illustrator, a naturalist, an animal behavior researcher, a city planner, a medical doctor, a blind social worker, a sound engineer, a child, and a dog. Each brought different features in the environment to Horowitz's attention.

- If you were to accompany Horowitz on a walk around a New York City block, what might capture your attention? What do you think you would share about what you notice on your stroll?
- Now turn your attention to the classroom. What do you tend to notice when you are teaching?

Clearly, Horowitz would have no book if we all saw the world the same way. Therefore, a book about the influence of what people notice seems like an apt reference to set the stage for *Part III*. Generally speaking, this last part focuses on how the exemplary teachers see and make sense of what they notice. It includes the final four chapters: Chapter 11, "Curiosity"; Chapter 12, "Reflection"; Chapter 13, "Preparation and Self-Care"; and Chapter 14, "What Makes Great Teachers Great?" and the appendixes.

- To begin, consider your teaching practice. What specific skills support your success? What personal practices positively influence your ability to be successful?

Chapter Eleven

Curiosity

In *The Hungry Mind*, Williams College's Susan Engel highlights how hard it is to adequately articulate curiosity's complexity. The internal urge of curiosity is "hitched to the outer world by way of thoughts concerning whatever event, information, or object an individual doesn't expect or understand."[1] This experience of curiosity is dynamic and multifaceted. It serves as a catalyst, spurring action.

Curiosity is powerful. It features a quality of confident, focused interest and enables learning by drawing attention to novel information, people, and situations.[2] According to Hulme, Green, and Ladd, high-curiosity students "tend to pursue uncertainty, exhibit openness to discovery, and perform better in school."[3] In this chapter, you will read about how curiosity's "urge to know more" affects and informs the exemplary educators' teaching practices and how it serves as an important source of energy.[4]

- In what ways does curiosity feature in your teaching practice?

In 1978, curiosity research pioneer Daniel Berlyne found that, when teachers intentionally aroused their students' curiosity, students would persist longer and with greater effort on the learning task, resulting in improved outcomes.[5] More recently, University of California, Davis, researchers used brain imagery to find that the reward and memory brain centers had heightened connectivity when study participants had an interest in the topic offered, leading to greater learning and recall of information. Once aroused, curiosity also had a positive effect on the learning and retention of topics of lesser interest.[6]

- From your experience, what does student curiosity look like and sound like?

Katie spoke about the power that teachers have to spark student curiosity: "If you like something, then you're excited about it—and if you're excited about it, the kids get excited about it." Curiosity is contagious. Teachers' curiosity levels spread to their students and influence educational outcomes.[7]

- Consider some examples when your curiosity spread to your students. What were some factors that caused that outcome?

Teachers who understand and value curiosity and the methods for curiosity's cultivation are better able to foster it in themselves and others, thereby creating the best possible learning environment for all.[8] A teacher's curiosity has the potential to inspire student imagination and cultivate an enduring passion for creating and pursuing meaningful questions and answers.[9]

Curiosity can be taught.[10] It is developable, but it requires educators' willingness "to embrace novelty and risk-taking" themselves.[11] Verbal and nonverbal educator modeling of curiosity is a powerful teaching tool. Examples of explicit teacher modeling of curiosity-based language include "I wonder what will happen when . . . ," "I really want to know why . . . ," and "I'm so curious about . . ." Two additional approaches that can alter student levels of curiosity are (1) the clear link of mistakes—failure—discovery, and (2) the sincere demonstration of inquiry into the unknown as a means to create an interesting and meaningful life.[12]

- What are some ways you model curiosity for your students?

CULTIVATING EXPERTISE

The exemplary educators have an understanding of their strengths as teachers, and through reflection they gain insight into how they achieve their successful educational outcomes. In short, they know what works for them. However, it is important to note, for the exemplary teachers in the study, their expertise is fluid.

Researchers Langer and Brookfield agree with this orientation, explaining how a fixed sense of expertise originating from past success-based habits, not mindfully applied, can lead to less-than-optimal outcomes.[13] An emphasis on cultivating expertise versus maintaining the status quo is a hallmark of the exemplary educators' approach to teaching.

- What are some ways you cultivate your expertise?

The exemplary teachers hold the presupposition that there is more than one right or best way to do things. They assume that positive alternatives to current practices exist. They also appreciate that all is not already known. Their approach to being a teacher aligns with Tangney's six key elements of humility:

1. the accurate assessment of one's abilities and achievement.
2. the ability to acknowledge one's mistakes, imperfections, gaps in knowledge, and limitations.
3. the openness to new ideas, contradictory information, and advice.
4. the keeping of one's abilities and accomplishments ... in perspective.
5. the relatively low self-focus ... while recognizing that one is but one part of the larger universe.
6. the appreciation of the value of all things, as well as the many different ways that people and things can contribute to our world.[14]

The teachers' preeminent priority of addressing the diverse needs of all students spurs the educators forward as they thoughtfully experiment with new approaches, pedagogies, and curriculum. Reflection about their experimentation helps support comprehensive understanding of lesson hits and misses. The important role that reflection plays is the focus of the next chapter.

The teachers anticipate that things will not work perfectly for all students. Because students have varying needs, the educators view lesson adaptation as part of the teaching role. This expectation influences their response to situations requiring some level of adaptation. Some of the teachers' remarks conveyed the need to find new teaching approaches as less of a burden and more of a quest or treasure hunt.

Barb emphasized the connection between educator openness and success: "I think you have to be [open]. . . . Teaching [and learning] to me is ongoing; it never stops. I'm always learning. When I stop learning, then I should stop teaching because I think a good teacher is open to everything as a positive, not a negative. . . . [It's] what *can I do*. . . . How can I look at [situations] in a different way?"

Some of the teachers seemed delighted when describing techniques they used, activities they found, stories they told, and modifications they made to address student learning needs. It is not always simple or easy. Kayla well represented the teachers' views when she said, "You have to be willing to do what will help the kid be successful."

The relationships the educators forge and the meaning they find in the role influences their experience. They referenced how satisfying it feels when they figure out what works for a student. Some spoke of how deeply they value the chance to watch a student move from confusion to clarity. For example, Jillian said,

> I love to see those moments [when] something finally clicks. . . . That's nice to see . . . Especially the struggling [students], when they finally get something, it's *really* nice to see that. And the [students] that don't give up. . . . That kind of brings you back . . . on the days when you want to tear your hair out—because that happens! . . . When they finally get it, you're like, "*Oh*, this is why I do what I do."

- Think of times when you noticed a student's shift from confusion to clarity. What were those experiences like for you?

CURRICULUM CHANGES AND STRESS

Harvard researcher Rosabeth Kanter states, "Nobody likes change when it's something that's done to us. But change that we think up or embrace on our own is different—*that* kind of change we never grow tired of."[15] In educational settings, school district administration personnel tend to make the final decisions about which curriculum will be taught in their system, although in some cases, teachers are asked to share their curriculum preferences before a curriculum is changed.

Patty expressed frustration about how curriculum changes are handled in her town. In the past, a group of teachers would gather together over the summer to collaboratively learn the new curriculum. They would also attend in-person professional development with curriculum developers and receive in-school support with experts. Now, the teachers are more often left on their own to learn new curriculum, and less time is set aside for collaboration about the content and materials.

In addition, some exemplary educators highlighted the frequency of curriculum changes as an influential variable that interfered with their ability to do their job well. It can sometimes be stressful and hard to stop teaching a curriculum that has worked well in favor of a new approach. To complicate matters, sometimes schools institute a number of curriculum changes simultaneously. Barb described how a curriculum can influence the effectiveness of her teaching:

> I think the ... curriculum itself affects how I teach. [I] may be not as productive as [I'd] like to be. . . . [I've found] in all the years [I've been] teaching [that] we keep changing the tool. . . . What happens is that I feel that I've accomplished [something with a curriculum], and I feel really good about [it], and [then] it switches. . . . I feel like I have a hold on it, and then it changes.

Researchers have found frequent changes can influence teacher interest in investing in a new initiative because there is a sense that it, too, will be short-lived. Over time, the overall experience can lead to change fatigue that dampens productivity and openness.[16]

The exemplary teachers may not be initially pleased upon hearing that they need to let go of a now-favorite curriculum that they have had a great deal of success with and worked hard to master. However, they attempt to approach the inevitable change with diligence, openness, curiosity, and flexibility. The exemplary teachers work hard to not apply preconceptions or decide in advance that things will fail.

Barb explained why she focuses on giving the new curriculum a chance. For her, the opportunity to teach content more effectively is too important to miss. She mentioned how teaching a specific topic has the potential to spark a lifelong interest in her students. Barb said, a student may decide "you know, *that's* what I love" after learning something new during one of her lessons. She went on to say, "I really, truly think teachers need to be open to anything. *Try it.* Don't have this preconceived idea [that] it's not going to work before you even tried it, you know? [Once] I had a colleague say to me, "Well, it's not going to work." I said, "Have you tried it?" She said, "No." . . . It may not [work], but if you don't try, you never know!"

- What helps you negotiate change?

Teaching requires a great deal of educator learning.[17] It is a complex and difficult profession. The exemplary teachers' tendency to approach change with applied curiosity may be a clue to their success. When faced with a challenge, curiosity supports a person's ability to use a grounded and focused sense of purpose and meaning to negotiate uncertainty and positively deal with the threat of failure.[18]

Learning something new in a short time frame within a high-accountability environment can be stressful. Larrivee describes how the educator's influential higher-level thinking is impaired when the stress response is induced, influencing teacher effectiveness.[19] The stress response occurs when people face a perceived threat or stressor. This ancient automatic human response involves the body overriding normal functioning of the brain's prefrontal cortex, narrowing focus and impairing higher-level thinking. The body does this as part of its preparation to flee, freeze, or fight.[20]

If the stress response occurs too frequently or for too long, it is a threat to human health, well-being, and performance. Matta and Singer agree that it is the appraisal of a situation that causes the stress response; it is not the situation itself. Feelings and thoughts occur as a result of human interpretations of events, and different people can feel or think differently about the same thing.[21] The degree to which stress is a positive or negative influence depends on the person experiencing it. Importantly, not all stress is harmful. Stress also enlivens and energizes. In fact, too little stress cultivates fatigue and boredom.[22]

Research indicates stress, even at high levels, has the potential to foster positive growth and development.[23] High stress potentially forges mental toughness, perspective shifts, enhanced priorities, closer relationships, greater awareness, and a heightened appreciation of life. It also provides an opportunity to call forth and experience personal qualities, like bravery, courage, tenacity, and persistence.

- In what ways might curiosity influence a teacher's experience of stress?

Barb explained how watching other successful educators experiment informs her teaching practice. This modeling of experienced colleagues has made a difference. She said,

> I think one thing I've learned from people that I've . . . respected . . . is they give it a try. It doesn't hurt. It doesn't cost you anything. It's just a moment in time. See if it works. . . . I think that's the biggest thing. If people and teachers in this profession want to be successful, they have to be open. They have to try. They have to experience [new things]. . . . I want to learn, and I want to share [with others], and it has to be that way for you to be successful. . . . You *have to* have an open mind-set to take things in and apply it or try it. . . .
>
> I think sometimes people think it's not going to work because [they think], "That's not how I teach."

- How would you characterize how you teach?

LESSON DESIGN, PACING, AND SELF-MANAGEMENT

Educators must teach a great deal of material within a limited time frame, and students do not respond to the material in a standardized way. In order to successfully deal with the stress that this challenging situation creates, Katie, June, and Kim spoke about the importance of "less is more." They referenced how curriculum pacing, a clear connection to meaning and purpose, and teacher self-awareness when talking affects student learning outcomes.

Katie spoke about resisting the significant pressure to quickly keep moving through her curriculum: "Less is more. I think that's key. I think that we have so much thrown at us that we are all like, 'I've got to get this done and this done and this done!' But you've got to slow down and do it so that [it's done] well."

June similarly spoke about how important it is for students to come to "see how everything fits together." Trying to do too much at once or too quickly can muddy that aim. In addition, helping students develop a clear rationale for learning the material—its value, meaning, and purpose—can affect student attention, motivation, and curiosity. June shared that she always explains to her students why they are learning something: "*Why* we do it . . . and [then] they get excited. . . . I want them to know, *always*, why we are doing it—*why*—and [how] that [skill or topic] is something . . . useful [for their lives]. When we learn a skill, why is that skill useful? . . . So [then] it just has [more] value to them. It's more authentic learning."

- Consider some specific times when a student's curiosity affected learning outcomes. What caused and sustained the student's curiosity?

Cultivating student curiosity also helps June with her classroom management. June said, "We do a lot of . . . partner [learning], where they go off on their own without me sitting there [with them]." If students are genuinely interested in what they are learning, it affects their behavior.

- In what ways might a student's curiosity level affect that student's behavior when learning with others?

Even though there is tremendous pressure to cover or deliver a great deal of required content, Kim spoke about how providing breaks can recharge curiosity and motivation when learning: "I try to do more brain breaks and moving . . . more transitions: a small lesson; transition to practice, whether it is independent or with a partner or in a small group; and then reconvene and discuss what's happened. Just try and keep them from getting stagnant."

Maintaining student interest and engagement is vital to Kim. With a smile, Kim also mentioned how helpful it is when she can remember the limits of student attention:

> As far as direct instruction, [there's limits to] their attention span. . . . I do find there are days when . . . I [*really* want to say], "If I could I have your attention for two more minutes," [but] they are gone. (laughs)
>
> [If I keep talking], . . . all that's going to happen is, I am going to get frustrated with them, [but it's] because *I am* the one who is not stopping talking! (laughs) Like [I'm] filibustering, you know? (laughs) . . . It's so hard, but luckily, they get it, and they know [me], and some days some of them will say to me, "I'm done." And [then] I'm like, "Okay, that's what I need to know." (laughs)

- What are some ways you manage your curriculum demands?
- What helps you foster and maintain student curiosity?

CREATING INTERESTING LESSONS

Not one of the educators loves everything they are required to teach. When faced with a curriculum or content area that is not their favorite, nearly all the educators spoke in some way about adapting it. Often, they augment the required content with aspects of other subjects that they are also required to teach that they find enjoyable.

Suzy explained that she sometimes uses her enjoyment of reading to students to make dull lessons interesting. For example, she decided to read a short, funny, and very descriptive story to her students to set up her required adjective lesson:

> We have all these incredible published writers that we can learn from! I go back to my favorite subject, which is reading, and I let the professionals help me. So if I want to teach how to use great adjectives, I will pull out [this incredible book]. . . . I *love* reading to children. . . . "Look at this expansive vocabulary! . . . Let's see if we can try and do something like that in our sentences today."

Although it reduces time if the lesson does not change from one year to the next, Kim described how it promotes teacher burnout or boredom. She gave an example of how she makes changes to her teaching of science experiments. Then she said, "I don't want to be one of those teachers that's just going through the motions because I feel like that becomes evident to the students. . . . You're that boring teacher that isn't making it fun for them. It might be a fun activity, but they're not going to get as much out of it [when you are just going through the motions]."

The educators take a variety of actions to keep their lessons fresh and interesting, such as asking for help from colleagues, using the web to find new things to try, referencing notes from past professional development sessions, engaging in frequent experimentation based on student needs and teacher interest, and joining online teacher groups outside of school to share ideas.

- What are some ways you keep your lessons fresh and interesting?

An orientation of openness and flexibility coupled with active researching and experimenting helps the educators find creative solutions. This approach to overcoming the challenges inherent in teaching is a point of pride for some. In their descriptions, the educators choose to shift the narrative about and the focus of the negative situation, thereby transforming difficulties into opportunities to apply curiosity and creativity.

- Which of your skills, attributes, and strengths supports your ability to find creative solutions?

CURIOSITY AS AN ENERGY SOURCE

The exemplary teachers want to keep learning and, as Patty put it, "stay current," so they can better achieve their goals as educators. Their desire to discover the unknown and create new knowledge is the essence of curiosity in action. Curiosity about what will happen when they try their new approaches focuses attention and creates energy.

According to Reio, curiosity's "related exploratory behaviors [such as] experimenting, consulting, reflection, and observing" positively affects human physical and psychological functioning.[24] Curiosity is an energizing force of openness and receptivity to new opportunities, discoveries, and meaning.[25] Research suggests that applied curiosity positively affects job performance, meaning and life satisfaction, and longevity.[26]

Curiosity fuels inquiry.[27] It has the potential to illuminate the previously unseen and unacknowledged via pursuit of purposeful intellectual, interpersonal, and intrapersonal exploration.[28] Jillian expressed the way curiosity acts as an energizing force:

> Every year is different, . . . and I like that. I implement . . . something new all the time. I am not afraid to change it. There are, of course, a couple of favorites that you go back to, but generally, I love trying new things. . . . Of course, there's [curriculum] . . . you have to do, but . . . [in this school] I do have [the] freedom to be a little bit more creative. . . . I am not afraid to try a new lesson, and I feel like I've got support [from the administration], too, which is nice. . . .
>
> Being able to try things, whether it's a lesson or fun things, . . . [like] today for math we assembled a [complicated] collaborative puzzle. [It was] something I've never done before, but my kids, they work so well together, [I thought I'd try it]. . . . To see them do that and kind of step back and watch them, I loved it.
>
> It does fail sometimes, and sometimes it works, but I think having something new every day [to try is important]. I have to look forward to [the lesson], too. If I am not looking forward to it, the [students] aren't going to look forward to it. . . . I think that element [of trying new things] makes me a stronger teacher. . . . I think that I learn with my kids. . . . It [also] makes me want to come to work.

The educators engage in ongoing reflection processes, and they know their students well, so their experimentation is not random; it is, instead, thoughtful, purposeful, and strategic. Because the educators recognize that the teacher brings the content and pedagogy to life, they work hard to create interesting lessons that address their students' needs. Importantly, the teachers spoke of the need to do things differently, not only for different students, but also for themselves.

- How does curiosity act as fuel for you?

Chapter Twelve

Reflection

According to Rachel, in order to be a successful teacher, you need to "be able to think on your feet. . . . You have to do it all day, every day." Thinking on your feet involves split-second conscious and unconscious brain processes affecting teacher noticing and interpreting and, ultimately, educational decision-making.[1]

Stanford Professor Emeritus Larry Cuban agrees, noting the improvisational nature of teaching and citing Philip Jackson's findings that "elementary teachers have 200 to 300 exchanges with students every hour (between 1200–1500 a day)." Jackson states, most of these exchanges are "unplanned and unpredictable calling for teacher decisions, if not judgments."[2]

- How do you know what to do when you need to think on your feet? What do you use to make those split-second decisions?
- What helps you make sound judgments?

This chapter explores: what the exemplary teachers use when they need to think on their feet; how their reflection practices affect and inform their teaching practices; and why the regularity of their reflective inquiry keeps their learning from experience fresh in their minds. This information yields an explanation of how the teachers' ongoing reflection updates their understanding of their personal best practices, affecting what they see, think, feel, and do when they need to think on their feet. As a starting point for this exploration of reflection, consider the following questions:

- What role does reflection play in your teaching practice?

- Generally speaking, what difference does reflection make when learning?
- In what ways can reflection influence memory?

EXPANDING REPERTOIRE AND ENHANCING UNDERSTANDING

Teaching is active. Throughout each day, teachers notice, interpret, and swiftly respond to what seems most important. Each person's understanding of life experience continually informs every situational response.[3]

According to Eberhardt, neuroscience research demonstrates that "our brains, our minds, are molded and remolded by our experiences and our environments. [In addition], we have the power to change our ways of thinking."[4] Executive brain functions allow us to gain insight into our thoughts, feelings, motives, behaviors, and desires.[5]

Practiced with regularity over time, reflection can create new mental habits that shape what a person notices. It also can affect how a person understands what has been noticed.[6] Deborah said, "I am very, very reflective. I think that that's a huge piece. [It's important to] think about your day and think about what worked and what didn't work and what you are going to do differently, whether it's [your] teaching, whether it's an individual student. You *have* to be reflective in teaching. I guess that's the biggest thing. You *have* to be reflective."

Reflection processes have tremendous potential for developing a person's self-awareness, self-management, social awareness, relationship skills, and responsible decision-making. However, reflection is just a tool. A tool's user affects the tool's effectiveness.

Many factors influence the depth, breadth, and accuracy of teacher reflection, such as current life events, emotional states, degree of curiosity, human developmental stages, change fatigue, relational-cultural interest, teacher knowledge base, the chosen reflection tool, adult social and emotional learning skills, and perceived time constraints. Humility can also play a role when reflecting. As highlighted in chapter 11, even though the exemplary teachers have had tremendous success, they each remain humble. They embrace that they are not perfect people or teachers. Because all is not already known, they assume there is something to learn every day. As Patty said, one key to teaching success is "you never stop learning."

This humble stance makes their time spent reflecting more productive. It also provides a rationale for engaging in processes of reflection. The meaning and purpose they find in the role and the quality of their teacher–student relationships fuels and informs their reflective inquiry.

- What fuels and informs your reflective inquiry?

Brookfield views teaching and learning as emotional, chaotic, and messy processes comprised of hard-to-resolve dilemmas.[7] The exemplary teachers use reflection to gain perspective, insights, and clarity. This habitual ongoing process broadens initial perceptions beyond first impressions.

When taking a second look, the teachers seek a dimensional cause-and-effect understanding. Through looking again at the situation, they end up with a deeper and more sophisticated grasp of what is happening in the classroom and why. They use this enhanced and updated understanding as the basis for future reactions and actions when, as Rachel put it, teachers need to "think on their feet."

- In what ways do your current reflection processes expand your repertoire and enhance your understanding when you need to think on your feet?
- What tends to be the focus of your reflection?

June expressed a strong interest in reflecting on practice, building skills, honing strategies, understanding teaching technique and student fit, and expanding repertoire. When reflecting, she considers both her teaching challenges as well as successes. For June, reflection is embedded in her way of being a teacher. She does not have a formal specific time or way of reflecting. She said, "I think we all, as good teachers, think about kids on the way home, . . . at home, or in the morning. . . . I think about . . . a moment that happened . . . the day before or a student or the lesson that *still* [doesn't] feel like it went well. . . . [It's important]. Be reflective—*always*."

June also pointed to the shelf in her classroom that contains past professional development materials. She keeps that learning alive by pulling out these materials periodically to refresh her memory of different approaches. She went on to say, "It's nice to have my toolbox, and it takes a while to build one, but then . . . [I] always [am ready] to kind of change gears . . . [for] certain [students]. [It's about] knowing what kids need and being respectful to the [students]. That's huge. . . . Keeping current, . . . staying knowledgeable, . . . doing a lot of reflecting, . . . and wanting to know more."

- What are some ways reflection helps you keep current?

Jillian shared how reflecting with other teachers was a vital component of her success. She spoke about the value of having a "strong support system." Jillian said, "A lot of my friends [outside of school] are teachers, as well. . . . You need that." She went on to describe how important it was for her to be able to talk over what happened during a school day

> because there are frustrations. Even [on] the most prepared day, it happens. . . . Without [my friends who are also teachers], I don't know how I'd make it and vice versa. We help each other out. . . . [We listen and discuss] the good or the bad, whatever needs to be said. We [really] do help each other. . . . I have a strong team here [in this school, as well], which is huge. We all work really nicely together, so all those pieces together help me feel better about my job.

- Do you have people with whom you regularly reflect? If so, how does that process support your ability to teach?

Barb feels similarly about the importance of reflection. It serves as the foundation of her teaching practice. She said, "I think the biggest key [to my success] . . . is reflection." She uses a variety of methods. She reflects on her own when running before school in the morning and also informally throughout the day. As mentioned in chapter 9, Barb regularly reflects with her highly valued classroom aide to learn what her aide notices, thinks, and feels about what is happening in the classroom. Her aide also provides Barb with feedback concerning the effectiveness of various teaching approaches. Barb's humility, openness, and curiosity make good use of her aide's second set of eyes. Another component of Barb's reflection process involves writing. Barb said,

> I was told at a very young age [that] journal writing is a powerful tool, and I journal write as a teacher. . . . I use those opportunities to reflect on my practice. . . . [In my journal] I have a section on each [student] in my room. . . . I see where they are, where I need to get them, what things worked that day or didn't work that day, and how I can do my best practices to get them where they need to be.
>
> [When things are not working as expected], I go back and write in my reflection journal. . . . How am I going to fix that, [as well as] why it didn't work, so that I can say, "Okay, what can I do differently next time?"

Barb's process of consistent journal writing can aid her overall understanding because over time both micro and macro views of what is occurring in the classroom can more clearly come into focus. This type of reflective inquiry can support dimensional understanding of the "dynamics of *when I do this, the consequence is that*, and how to use these insights to change the system for the better."[8] It can also create a more sophisticated appreciation of the interdependence of the individual elements that work together to create outcomes.[9]

According to Senge and colleagues, humans have a problematic tendency to deeply consider what is familiar while also maintaining a blindness to influential variables that can be larger in scope or not immediately self-serving.[10] Goleman and Senge explain, "Systems operate everywhere . . . [although] we may not be aware of . . . how we are shaped by them—and shape them in return."[11] Reflective inquiry has the potential to expand the scope of variables under consideration when problem-solving, which can, in turn, result in the emergence of different solutions to complex challenges.[12]

- What are some strategies you use to comprehend both the "big picture" and "small picture" views of what is happening in your classroom?

Interestingly, researchers have found the use of writing processes, like Barb's practice, can promote overall health and well-being during difficult and stressful experiences.[13] Challenging situations tend to narrow attentional focus. They can foster rumination that serves as a distraction during the day and can disrupt sleep at night. Researchers at the Greater Good Science Center at the University of California, Berkeley, state, "Expressive writing allows us to step back for a moment and evaluate our lives. Through writing, we can become active creators of our own life stories—rather than passive bystanders—and as a result feel more empowered to cope with challenges. Transforming a messy, complicated experience into a coherent story can make the experience feel more manageable."[14]

Larrivee highlights how adopting a consistent writing practice also allows teachers to enhance their awareness of the ways they contribute to their experiences. In addition, it can help teachers gain or renew their sense of meaning and purpose. Discovering personal meaning is a key variable for burnout prevention.[15]

- What are some ways you cultivate your sense of meaning and purpose?
- How do you reflect?
- How does reflection help?

One benefit of teacher reflection is the illumination of what affects the quality of teacher–student relationships. Many patterns of social interaction arise through ingrained habitual behavior. Each of us has powerful habits, beliefs, and biases that act on the conscious and unconscious levels.[16]

In *Biased: Uncovering the Hidden Prejudice That Shapes What We See, Think, and Do*, Eberhardt describes how

> racial bias affects all sorts of decisions we make during the normal course of our lives—the homes we buy, the people we hire, the way we treat our neighbors. Bias is not limited to one domain of life. It is not limited to one profession, one race, or one country. It is also not limited to one stereotype association. . . . Neither our evolutionary path nor our present culture dooms us to be held hostage by bias. Change requires a kind of open-minded attention that is well within our reach.[17]

Through intentional processes of inquiry, current ways of seeing, thinking, feeling, and behaving can become more apparent. Once bias is identified and understood, teachers become better positioned to create more equitable learning experiences.[18] Eberhardt states, "there is hope in the sheer act of reflection. This is where the power lies and how the process starts."[19]

- What are some strategies you have used to increase your awareness of your biases?

The school administration plays an important role in Benson and Fiarman's developmental approach to addressing unconscious bias in school settings. They state, "What leaders say and pay attention to gets noticed. Equally important, however, are the topics we as leaders ignore, the issues around which we remain publicly silent."[20] They further explain, "We're all influenced by bias. Let's have the courage to face this and help reduce the effects of this bias on students. Let's not hide our blind spots but help each other see and address them. Let's be brave together. . . . Brave communities don't just happen. Leaders deliberately build them."[21]

Should you want to delve more deeply into this and related topics, please see the links to information and tools in appendix F under Bias, Implicit Cognition, and Educational Equity. The standpoint theory exploration included in appendix D may also be helpful.

ACQUIRING, REMEMBERING, AND APPLYING LEARNING FROM EXPERIENCE

When faced with a baffling teaching challenge, Barb shared that she examines her rich supply of teaching memories to try to come up with a solution. She spoke about accessing "prior experience, . . . and it could be [from] 10 years ago [when] I've had a [similar] kid." She feels such satisfaction when she remembers what worked before with other students. She says to herself, "This [just] might work! And [then when I try it], . . . *wow!* It worked!"

Suzy also highlighted how ready access to past learning from experience boosts her confidence and enhances the effectiveness of her teaching practice:

> From experience, I know that students who have this typically need to do this. And students who have this might typically need to do that. . . . I guess we all have our tool belts, with our tricks. . . . You just try one, and if that doesn't work, you pull out another one. (laughs) But you don't stop trying. . . . Now no one [student] fits the mold, but fortunately I have . . . experience, and I am able to apply that, and it does help. . . . It [also] helps with my confidence.

- What helps you remember what you have learned from experience so you have access to it when you need it?

One way to remember learning from experience is through a regular process of reflective inquiry; frequency matters. According to Memory Lab director and Washington University psychology professor Roddy Roediger, retrieving knowledge makes memories stronger. Roediger states, "We don't get information into memory just to have it sit there. We get it in to be able to use it later. . . . The actual act of retrieving the information over and over, that's what makes it retrievable when you need it. . . . Memory is dynamic, and it keeps changing, . . . and retrieval helps it change."[22]

Importantly, each time a memory is retrieved, it then becomes linked to new contexts and sensations: "The more things you have it connected to, the easier it is to pull it out, because you have lots of different ideas that can lead you to that particular material. . . . And the things you retrieve get more accessible later on, and the things you don't retrieve get pushed into the background and become harder to retrieve next time."[23] Therefore, when teachers regularly reflect, they set themselves up to learn and remember what works, what does not work, and why. This continually updated dimensional understanding of teaching and learning becomes what teachers use when they need to think on their feet.

- How has reflection consistency influenced your ability to remember and deepen your learning from experience?
- Have you ever attended a thought-provoking one-day professional development workshop about a new educational approach? If so, in what ways did your consideration (or lack of further consideration) of the workshop learning affect your ability to remember and apply the new approach in the days and weeks after the workshop?
- What are some strategies you use to transform an initial personal insight into a desired long-lasting, substantive change?

THE GLASS IS HALF-EMPTY AND HALF-FULL

One skill Wanda thinks helps support her teaching success is her capacity to reflect about what is good in situations as well as the more obvious problems and challenges. Wanda said, "You know what it is. . . . It's finding the positivity in every day."

As highlighted in chapter 9, the exemplary teachers, like all humans, have a negativity bias that makes the negative in situations easier to notice, remember, and relive.[24] However, it is possible for the metaphorical glass to be construed as being both half-empty and half-full. For example, people can develop fault-finding, benefit-finding, and strength-finding skills. Being able to see both the good and the bad within a circumstance, along with feeling both the corresponding positive and negative emotions, requires emotional agility, expands situational understanding, and increases well-being.[25]

When reflecting, the exemplary teachers thoughtfully consider problem situations and teaching challenges. However, they also strive to seek out, appreciate, and reflect about successes, as well. Through this approach to reflection, teachers can end up with a clearer picture of what they can do, as well as what to avoid.

Teaching is personal. An approach that works well for one teacher may be less effective for another. For each teacher, reflection can foster better understanding of the causes and effects of their successful and unsuccessful teaching efforts and outcomes. It can help teachers create a complex and personalized understanding of "my best practices."

- How has reflecting about what works and what does not helped you refine your personal best practices?

BENEFITS OF APPRECIATING SUCCESSES

Understanding how and why successes occurred is valuable. As Suzy and Barb explained, it helps them develop a broader understanding of what has worked for them with different students, making their current teaching practices and educational interventions more effective. In addition, when teachers share the positive information gleaned from reflection on successes, it can affect other people's positivity. For example, reflection about and comprehensive understanding of a successful teaching outcome may yield a greater appreciation of how hard particular students worked to learn something new. The teacher then can follow up with students one-on-one, pointing out the specific application of skills, qualities, or attributes that caused their learning outcome. The celebration of student effort fosters teacher and student positivity.

- Think of a time when you celebrated a hard-won success with a student. What was that experience like for you? What might your student have been thinking and feeling?

As mentioned in earlier chapters, the teachers also want positive information to share and celebrate with their students' parents and caregivers. To that end, the teachers are on the lookout for examples of academic successes or qualities like perseverance, helpfulness, or kindness. Reflection about successes is one source for that information.

As Kayla said, "There *has to be* something nice you can say about *any child* to a parent. It's their baby." She went on to share how a parent said to her, "'Thank you so much! Last year's teacher *never* said a positive. It was *always* negative,' and I said, 'But it's not *all* negative. There are some behaviors that are negative, but it's because of his issue.' . . . You have to see that children aren't *bad*. There are things that cause them to do things, . . . and you have to be willing to help them."

- How have parents or caregivers responded when you shared something positive about their child?

Through reflection of what works, teachers may also become more aware of other people's contribution to their success, spurring gratitude and thankfulness. Thanking, savoring, and celebrating with close colleagues nurtures the collegial bond and spreads positivity. It can also strengthen relational trust, highlighted in chapter 10 as a foundational school success variable. Understanding what works well can act as an energy source between teachers, supporting collective educator efficacy and well-being.

- What helps nurture collegial bonds in your school?
- In what ways does your understanding of past teaching successes positively affect your current teaching practice?

Barb concisely presented the exemplary educators' views: "I'm a big believer in positive reflection, [and] positive energy gives positive results." The teachers want to remember positive teaching moments and understand what caused them.

Frenzel, Goetz, Stephens, and Jacob's found "teachers' emotions have a reciprocal influence on their instructional behavior . . . which in turn influences student outcomes."[26] Importantly, greater awareness and appreciation of successes can foster an upward spiral of positivity that acts as a buffer to negative experience and supports greater resilience.[27] According to Fredrickson, "Positive emotions . . . trigger broadened, curious, and optimistic patterns of thought together with more spontaneous and energetic behavior. These thought-action tendencies increase the odds that people find positive meaning in their future circumstances in ways that seed further positive emotions that decrease stress, provide emotional uplift, and support resilience."[28]

- Think of some examples when your positive emotions (e.g., gratitude, interest, inspiration, amusement, pride, joy, serenity, love, awe, hope) influenced your behavior. What were you feeling? What did you do or say? What were some possible effects on others?
- What are some approaches you use to reflect on what works well?

It is important to note that reflection processes can serve as a vehicle for cultivating hope in an ongoing way. Reflection can provide an opportunity to reconnect with meaningful goals. It can enhance appreciation of inner resources and outside supports (agency thinking). It also can help expand awareness of multiple paths forward (pathway thinking).[29] To learn more, review chapter 9 and see appendix E.

Chapter Thirteen

Preparation and Self-Care

Much of teaching involves observation and sophisticated analysis of that which has been seen. According to Louis Pasteur, a founder of microbiology, "In the fields of observation, chance favors only the prepared mind."[1] In this chapter, the exemplary teachers' share how self-care and other preparation practices influence what they notice and also what they think, feel, and believe about what they have seen.

- What are some of your current self-care and preparation practices?

FEELING READY

Katie smiled broadly when she identified the first two keys to her feeling ready to teach: "coffee and sleep!" She went on to further explain other aspects of her preparation process, saying with a laugh, "I am a crazy person with my lesson plans. My team makes fun of me. . . . [My plans] are *so* elaborate, it's crazy, and [I know] I'm a little over the top." Katie then gestured to different places in the classroom while further explaining how she "preps" for the next day:

> My objectives are already written for tomorrow. My morning message is already written for tomorrow. [That] work (points to a pile of materials) will be on [each students'] desk for the morning before I leave [today], so that when I come in [tomorrow], I can concentrate on lesson plans for next week or maybe [make] phone calls home [to parents. Or I could use that time to be] grading something or planning an activity. . . .

> I just feel like if you're prepared, that's half the battle. Because, if you're not prepared, [students] are going to eat you alive. . . . They are going to take that 3 minutes of unstructured time [that it took you to prepare yourself] to maybe argue with somebody next to them, fool around, [or whatever], and then your day is like *ugh*. It snowballs! So [preparation's] *huge*.

- What are some things that you do to prepare yourself and your classroom for a day of teaching?

Patty's remarks were similar to Katie's. However, to Patty, being prepared well in advance is an act of self-care because it reduces the anxiety that can arise from having to manage all the details that come with teaching. In addition to getting a "good night's sleep," Patty said,

> I am a very organized person. . . . I can't fly by the seat of my pants [and feel] ready for the day. . . . I need to prepare materials . . . [because] a lot of these things are hands-on and there's a lot of things required to get those activities in place, so you can't leave it for the day before. . . .
>
> I feel like I am mentally ready when I feel good about having everything in order. . . . I am someone that does things in advance, *well* in advance, because I don't want to wait (e.g., reports, projects, IEP meeting planning, report cards). . . . That's too anxiety provoking for me. . . . I want to be done with it and move on to the next thing. I don't want that hanging over me, you know? . . . I am prepared and ready to go if I feel healthy and rested and I've done what I have to do to start the day.

Barb also mentioned health. Her preparation processes are informed by her strong interest in being healthy and modeling healthiness for her students:

> Healthiness gives you strength to do what you need to do each day. [It's] taking care of your body, your mind, and your soul each day. I always say, "If I can do something for my mind, body, and soul each day, I'm going to be a better person, and I'm going to be a better teacher," so I think those things play a big part in what [happens] in the classroom. . . .
>
> There's a couple things I do [to prepare]. . . . I'm a runner, so every morning . . . I run, and I think. I run by myself, and I think every day. . . . I get my mind set for my day. So that's my physical part that I do. . . . Then I come in with the concept of being [and] focusing on the positive-ness of the day and being mindful of what can happen each moment. So, that's how . . . I prepare myself. I'm ready to go every day . . . and ready to see what the day brings.

- What helps you feel ready for a day of teaching?

Rachel shared that she does not ever really feel fully prepared and ready for a day of teaching:

> I don't know a teacher that can say "I am 100% prepared for today" because you don't know what is walking in the classroom. You know the kids, [but] you don't know what they are going to do when they come into the classroom. They can be great kids every day you have ever known them, [but] . . . maybe they woke up 2 minutes ago, and they're flustered, or maybe a grandparent died [or something else happened] that you don't know.
>
> So, I don't think teachers can ever be prepared enough. . . . I write my lesson plans out, and I [work hard to] make sure I get [things] done, . . . [but] things get in the way, meetings happen, kids get called out, [students] get dismissed. I mean, things happen. . . . I think attempting to be prepared is very important because it helps you keep on track, but you have to be able to roll with the punches. If you're not a person who can do that, [then] this is *not* the job for you! (laughs)

- What strengths, skills, and personal attributes do you have that support your ability to negotiate the unexpected that comes with each day of teaching?

PREPARATION, SUPPORT, AND TEACHING'S EARLY YEARS

June emphasized how hard it was when she was a new teacher. The amount of learning and preparation required for just one day of teaching for a new teacher is significant. June described how "at this point, I know the skills I am teaching. I know the material I am teaching. But I remember years ago, having to bring things home, and . . . it was like I was doing a final every night! Studying social studies, studying how they did the math problems for the next day—it was a lot of work!"

Katie's sentiments, though similar to June's, emphasized the additional challenges new teachers face today: "I feel so bad for [new teachers] because . . . it [is] *so much* harder now, with all the . . . Common Core, the high-stakes testing, and just the everyday craziness of teaching—parents, . . . kids, and the way children socialize or don't socialize enough. There's not enough time for them to learn how to play. They're always on technology. There's so many things!"

Deborah also spoke about how preparation processes change with experience and how complex teaching is for new teachers:

I know what I have to teach like the back of my hand. So, my time isn't spent learning Chapter 3, Unit 4, Week 1. My time is spent on my kids because I don't have to focus so much on *what* I am teaching or *how*. . . .

I think [during] the first few years, [it can feel like] you're like swimming upstream, learning [all the] curriculum. You're [also] learning how to deal with different colleagues. You're learning who to trust in the building—who to confide in—when you screw something up, you know? You're learning. [It's like], "Oh my gosh, I can't find those copies that I ran off that I'm supposed to [use for] that lesson right now, and I am so afraid somebody's going to come through the door!" That's the mind-set of a first-year teacher.

It takes a lot of support, and they're going to fall. . . . It's a matter of supporting them and just saying, "You know, we've all been there. We've all been those new young teachers thrown into a classroom and still responsible for [everything related to student] learning."

Jillian described how she negotiated the uncertain and changeable nature of her early years teaching:

I know . . . a lot of people [who went through something similar]. . . . You get bumped from your grade level, [and there's no job security]. I looped with my kids. . . . I moved schools. Every year, I had a fresh start. I had to start from scratch. I just took it in stride. I had a job. I was [doing] what I love to do. It's okay that I'm not perfect every year because, you know, there is no such thing. . . .

By going through those experiences and just being patient with it, I knew I'd end up where I wanted to be. . . . [All the changes] kind of comes with the territory. . . . Until you're permanent [and have job security], you kind of have to go with it. . . . It's important to rely on [colleagues], and you [really] do have to understand [that] you know more than you think [and] . . . have confidence [in] yourself. . . . And you have to have that mind-set that it's okay and that you can teach anything. . . .

[School] can't consume you. The first couple of years, it does and that's normal, but as I [have] kind of [been] growing in my teaching experience, I [now] know that it's okay to have an outside life. You *do* have to separate it, and you *do* have to take time for yourself.

While it is clear that Jillian found a way to negotiate the challenges that come with being a new teacher, teacher attrition is a significant challenge in education.[2] Having experienced and well-qualified teachers influences educational outcomes.[3] According to Greenberg, Brown, and Abenavoli, four programs that have been "proven to help teachers reduce stress, improve wellbeing and students outcomes, and even save schools money [are] . . . mentoring/induction programs, . . . workplace wellness programs, . . . social emotional learning programs, . . . and mindfulness/stress management programs."[4]

Deborah highlighted the value of formal and informal mentorship of novice teachers. As a mentor in the state-mandated mentoring program, Deborah is randomly paired with a new teacher. However, Deborah thinks the school administration also should support more informal novice-veteran teacher connections:

> I know that [having informal mentors] was what worked for me. I had some really good role models in [my early years], and to this day, I still go back to some of the things I learned from them. . . . I am still very close to one of them I met during my first year out of [college. She is now retired]. . . . I learned *everything* from her. I think that that relationship taught me a lot about not only just teaching and curriculum and reading but also about loving the kids. . . . She knows it. I tell her all the time, . . . "I learned everything from *you!*"

- What or who helped support your development as a teacher?
- What or who helps you grow now?

BEING MINDFUL

When there is a significant outside stressor, Katherine works hard to prepare herself for a day of teaching by being especially mindful and self-aware. She spoke about the importance of setting aside any outside upset, whether a personal situation, like ill health, or a professional issue, like a before-school disagreement with a colleague about the level of student services needed.

Katherine highly values the positive and productive relationships she creates with each student. She also shared that some of her students have challenges that significantly tax her patience. As a result, Katherine recognizes that she needs to prepare herself well, so she can treat her students with the respect they deserve. She said, "In kindergarten, you can't afford not to have the patience that you need. . . . [For example] I have a child who . . . needs things repeated to him a number of times, rephrased a number of different ways, . . . and [it's really hard] when you don't feel well or you've had a really bad discussion with [the speech teacher or reading teacher] before the kids come in." To ready herself, Katherine sometimes focuses on her breathing, or she mindfully savors a cup of coffee "You have to just, like, take a breath. (pause) Have a cup of coffee (pause). A nice, hot, cup of coffee. You have to relax."

In this example, Katherine uses the mindfulness practice of intentionally shifting her attention to the present moment through noticing her breath or tending to her enjoyment of the coffee she drinks. Through the change of the focus of her attention—the intentional pause and the positive experience of savoring and appreciating her coffee—Katherine gains increased calm. The recalibration supports a more compassionate and thoughtful response imbued with the patience that Katherine views as crucial for her teaching success.

Smalley and Winston suggest that mindfulness practices like those described by Katherine act to clean the lens of our experience and foster a better understanding of how personalized filters affect perception, feeling, and thinking.[5] Cultivating mindful awareness can foster a bigger picture view of circumstances. This different perspective supports insight into and a broader understanding of situational factors and conclusions regarding available options; "Instead of [just] giving into one's usual conditioned, habitual behavior, [mindful awareness can give people] . . . a greater sense of freedom and choice."[6]

Relatedly, one of the possible benefits of consistent contemplative practice is reduced reactivity and enhanced well-being.[7] According to Goleman and Senge, "Just as the perception of danger generates adrenaline and focuses attention on immediate possible sources of threat, so too does [our] ability to slow down and be more aware of our larger settings—internally and externally—develop when we feel safe and learn how to access a more holistic awareness of the present moment."[8]

When Katherine brings the student who requires multiple explanations to mind, she thinks to herself, "It's not his fault, you know. (pause) He has a processing issue." Through that method she is able to connect with her compassion for her student, renewing her supply of patience. Being mindful helps Katherine prepare herself well for her teaching day. For additional research-based information and tools, please see the Mindfulness, Compassion, and Gratitude section in appendix F.

- What are some strategies you use when negotiating a relationship with a student who tries your patience?

Later, Katherine went on to reference extremely challenging times, such as being sleep deprived due to her daughter's illness. She said, teaching "can be very stressful . . . —really joyous, too, and rewarding—but it also can be extremely stressful when . . . you are going through something really hard." In those situations, Katherine knows she is not at her best, so she reaches out to close colleagues and asks for help. Sometimes, all Katherine needs is an extra minute or two to compose herself. Her colleague will say, "Just go make yourself a cup of coffee, and then come back." Being able to lean on colleagues for support makes *such* a difference for Katherine.

- How might having close relationships with colleagues influence Katherine's sense of readiness to handle what comes during a day of teaching?

EMBRACING IMPERFECTION

Despite her best efforts, Suzy still misjudges her readiness on occasion. She relayed a time during the previous week when her adverb lesson was not successful due to ineffective preparation:

> It was my fault. I wasn't 100% prepared to teach them adverbs, and . . . I own it—I absolutely own it. I didn't have my chart ready, . . . so I was trying to draw it on the fly. I [realized the lesson wasn't working], . . . and I shut it down right in the middle, and I apologized. I said, "You know what, boys and girls? I'm not prepared to teach this to you the way it should be taught to you. I am going to stop [the lesson], and I hope you don't mind." They were like, "Okay," and I said, "We're revisit this next week, and I promise, I'll be prepared."
>
> It doesn't happen often. I am a little bit of a type A, and I like to make sure everything is planned out and prepared. . . . I've got my charts [ready], and I know what I want to say. But it happened, and it happens.

Kayla also referenced mistakes, sharing how she is explicit about making mistakes in her classroom. She clearly tells her students that she does not expect them to be perfect: "I say to my kids, 'You use a pencil in math for a reason.' I make mistakes during the day. I expect them to make mistakes. I [say to them], '*That's* how we learn.'"

- What are some ways you highlight the role mistakes play in learning?

Debbie spoke about how being kind to herself was helpful, especially when things do not go perfectly during a day of teaching:

> I think [being kind to ourselves] is something we could all do more. I think that I can be kind to myself by allowing myself to say, "You know what? You made a mistake, and it's okay. You're human," and just move on. . . . I think that teachers can be very stressed. . . . Being able to give yourself an opportunity to just relax and . . . do for you—I don't think it is something that we do enough.

Debbie's ideas about being kind to herself along with her comment "You're human" align with some of the self-compassion recommendations mentioned in chapter 9. University of Texas, Austin, self-compassion researcher, Kristin Neff offers a variety of free research-based approaches that can be accessed via the Self-Compassion exercises link under the Mindfulness, Compassion, and Gratitude section in appendix F.[9]

- What are some ways you are kind to yourself?

Katie spoke about how it is not easy to embrace her imperfect attempts to balance all the responsibility that comes with such an important job. The pressure is stressful. Katie said, "I think it's a big role. . . . I think we put a lot of pressure on ourselves, and I think sometimes we need to be like, 'Okay, you're doing a lot. (laughs) Take a break, you know? Give yourself some credit.' . . . I think we need to take a little bit of the pressure off ourselves sometimes, which is hard. I mean, you want the best for the school, for the kids, for the class, so [it's hard]."

Jillian shared an example of her attempt to balance caring for her health and meeting the demands of the job. Although she regularly grades and returns student work promptly, Jillian said there have been times when "you will be grading, [and it's] 10:00 at night. . . . Sometimes, you have to call it [quits]—and if the kids don't get their papers back for a week, they don't get it back for a week." While this delay is atypical for Jillian and it is not ideal, it has happened.

- What helps you balance all the responsibility that comes with such an important job?

Kim also referenced how complicated a personal and professional life balance can be:

> It is important to make time for yourself, so you're not feeling burnt out, . . . especially if it's a tough year, . . . even a tough week, sometimes. [You]

definitely need to find things to do that you enjoy because on those tough days you need to have something, so . . . I'd definitely say [that's] important. But, you know, . . . there's a line. There's the balance between worrying too much about yourself and your own personal life because if you are . . . worrying so much about your outside life, . . . you are not going to be doing your best [here].

- What are some ways you negotiate work demands and your life outside school?

Suzy offered an additional perspective. She described how her work helps her when she is experiencing challenges in her personal life: "It's almost the beauty of teaching. Regardless of what's happening out there in our personal lives, you *have to* leave it at the door because these little people, . . . they are all over you, and the beauty of it is, if [I am] having a rough time of it outside [school], I find I can't worry about it until I leave. (laughs) I can't even *think* about it until I leave."

- How might Suzy's commitment to fostering positive teacher–student relationships, coupled with the meaning and purpose she finds in the teaching role, inform and affect her ability to shift her focus and leave outside worries "at the door"?

FOCUSING ENERGY ON WHAT CAN BE INFLUENCED

Every exemplary teacher referenced the significant challenges facing educators today, such as too much curricula, testing, and paperwork and too little time, support, and funding. Teaching requires significant personal, emotional, and intellectual efforts, moment by moment and throughout every day.[10] The educators expressed frustration with much of what happens in education.

They all shared examples of their openness and flexibility when negotiating the unexpected and unwanted that consistently affect their lives as teachers. A hallmark of the educators is their ongoing intentional attempts to focus on accepting what they have no power to change. Instead, they emphasize putting tremendous effort into what they can influence. Three expressly stated how they just have to "make it work."

Katherine spoke about how important it is for teaching success to reach out to colleagues for support. She also emphasized the value of self-awareness and self-management during teacher–teacher conversations because it can be hard to not focus on the unchangeable negative: "When you have other teachers who are excellent . . . and you put . . . your heads together, . . . it makes a difference. . . . [However], you do *really* have to try, *really* hard not to let the negative . . . get into your head . . . because it can bring you down. . . . You just have to get back to the basics of what you are here for."

Katherine's suggestion is not always easy to put into action because, as mentioned elsewhere, the negative in situations tends to stand out and grab our attention.[11] This negativity bias is a natural aspect of human perception. It supported species survival. Negative situational features that are clearly and vividly remembered are also more likely avoided in the future.[12] That does not mean the positive has little value, although sometimes it may feel that way.

- When having conversations with colleagues, what supports your ability to set aside the negative such that you are able to focus your energy on what can be influenced?

As Rachel said, even though she may really want to, "pouting about it" will not change anything. Often "there is no way around it." The exemplary educators work hard to find a way to move through the negative and be positive. For example, Kayla developed a system with family members that she gets five minutes to vent (without using any names or other identifiers), and then they need to help her move on. The focus on acceptance of the unchangeable affects where teachers choose to place their attention and how they choose to expend their precious and limited energy.

- What helps you manage unchangeable teaching challenges?

PREPARING THE SELF BROUGHT TO TEACHING

Kerry Howells of the University of Tasmania describes how people have highly influential inner attitudes, whether tended to or not. The inner attitude that each teacher holds before an event influences what ultimately happens. Therefore, Howells suggests educators not only prepare lesson content and pedagogy each day but also the states of being that they are bringing to their teaching. Howells references Palmer's notion *teachers teach who they are* when she invites educators to thoughtfully explore the *I* in the statement *I teach who I am.*[13] Nieto expresses similar sentiments: "Teachers bring their entire autobiographies with them: their experiences, identities, values, beliefs, attitudes, hangups, biases, wishes, dreams, and hopes. It is useless for them to deny this; the most they can do is acknowledge how these may either get in the way of, or enhance, their work with students."[14]

Debbie shared how her self-knowledge affects lesson planning:

> I know if I am not in a good mood [and] . . . if I'm particularly stressed that the things that my [students] do can be a little bit more (pause). . . . I can be more reactive to them, . . . so . . . if I had something planned that day, . . . [and] I can tell that . . . I am not in the right place for it, sometimes I might just change it. . . . I try to be really mindful of . . . how my attitude can be clouding my perception of what [my students] are doing.

Debbie and the other exemplary teachers are very aware of their emotional states and manner at school. In fact, some demonstrated understanding of emotional contagion by discussing how teacher negativity can spread to students and colleagues (see chapter 10). They take responsibility for how they are feeling and, using self-awareness and self-management, respond accordingly.

They use a variety of strategies to sustain themselves over the course of the year. They have a personal network of support (e.g., family, friends, pets) and renewing self-care processes (e.g., exercise at the gym, hiking in the woods, time in the mountains, gardening in the yard, caring for pets, organizing gatherings, pursuing hobbies). For example, Jillian said,

> You do need to take that time for yourself, whether it's a walk or a manicure or a whatever it is, [like] going out with a friend for dinner. You need to do it. . . . Outside of school, I take my dog for little walks, so that's a huge thing—exercise. My family and my friends, they're all . . . very close in distance, so I'm always over at their houses . . . just to have that outside life as well [as] school.

The exemplary teachers put forth a great deal of effort to manage themselves such that they spread authentic positivity throughout their classrooms. It could be just remembering to notice and tend to the cultivation of positive teacher–student and student–student relationships. Other times, it could be creating opportunities for the class to laugh together, whether through reading a funny book together or watching a comical one-minute video as a class.

Some educators place reminders of their past positive teaching experiences within easy view. These personal mementos take a variety of forms (student-created artwork, letters from past students, framed photographs of students). These visual reminders nurture and strengthen positive memories. Other educators post inspirational quotes or poems on the wall or near the teacher's desk as visual cues to foster educator positivity. For example, Suzy shared how important it was to remember

> What an impact I can have on these [students]! . . . I have got these quotes (points to the wall). I try to read them every day—"I have come to a frightening conclusion I am the decisive element in this classroom. It is my personal approach that creates the climate. It's my—*I love this*—it is my daily mood that makes the weather, and I . . . possess tremendous power to make a child's life miserable or joyous," and on and on it goes.
>
> We have such an incredible impact on these [students]. We can make them or break them! And when you get [a student] who comes back and says, "Look at who I am, in part, because of you"—*Wow!*

- What are some things you do to support yourself over the course of the year?
- What are some ways you spread authentic positivity in your classroom?

WHAT IS RECEIVED?

In contrast to a focus on what is wrong and what is lacking, applied gratitude invites consideration of what also exists that is good and helpful. To Howells, gratitude is, in part, an expression of thanks toward another person.[15] It is embedded within a relational context. Due to the interpersonal relationship between teacher and student, gratitude can play a role in teaching.

Lyubomirsky, Kurtz, Watkins, Howells, and others assert that gratitude practices are not a one-size-fits-all short-term solution. Instead, gratitude is a vehicle for growth through reflection.[16] By deeply savoring what is good and what is working, a greater appreciation of what is happening can emerge. Should you want to learn more about gratitude practices, please see the research-based information in the Mindfulness, Compassion, and Gratitude section in appendix F.

Howells found that teacher gratitude cultivation methods positively affected educator "presence, efficacy, and resilience."[17] The teachers working with Howells were able to move from a more narrow consideration of what they were not getting from students to intentionally noticing and considering the positive they were receiving from students.

With Howells' gratitude research in mind, the exemplary teachers were asked what they receive from being a teacher and what they receive from their students. As soon as one question was asked, some teachers immediately teared up; they answered with words like *joy* and *laughter*. Suzy described how the job provides the opportunity to make a difference in people's lives every day: "To know that I have actually encouraged someone to try something [new], to be bigger than they thought they could be, to be better than they thought they could be—what an incredible gift! I feel so blessed to be here and have this job and have this opportunity *every day*."

Deborah also referenced how she receives something from teaching every day:

> Every single day . . . gives me something—*every single day*! It is one of the most rewarding things, other than being a parent. It's so rewarding! Like one of my [students]—it clicked—he's reading! *That's* so rewarding to me. I'm like, *oh my god*, he's got it! . . .
>
> Or maybe [it's] that you know [a student] spent the weekend with her dad and she loved it, and she came in Monday and was as happy as could be. You know, *that's* rewarding. . . . [It's] knowing that she's okay. . . . She understands now [what's happening with her family, and] she's going to be okay. . . .
>
> [Also, when] they come back to visit, *that's* rewarding to me. [Or] when I am, you know, in Stop and Shop, and a 17-year-old kid comes over and says, "Hey—oh my god, . . . how are you? I saw you walking your dog the other day!" . . . [When students stop and want to talk], it's amazing. . . . You know you've made a difference in their life.

Kim described how she savors the gratitude she feels about being able to be a teacher:

> I have become very proud when I see successes or . . . [when] a parent says to me, "My child had a really good year" . . . because the teachers that I connected with as a child . . . made me *love* going to school. I just thought [school] was wonderful, [so] you really . . . can't beat that.
>
> I like the fact that I enjoy coming to work every day. There's so many people that just go through the motions . . . of their careers, or they'll call it their job. . . . It's just what they do because it's a means to an end. . . . I feel grateful that I can sit here (slowly looks around the room)—I remember having this moment, one of my first years teaching. I was like, "*Ahhhh!* Look at this! If this was my office, [I'd] have a *huge* office. (laughs) . . . I might share it with a bunch of little bodies, but it's mine."

And there's a lot of faith and trust in me that I'm going to be doing my job.... Somebody is not micromanaging constantly.... They've entrusted me to make sure that these [students] are successful [and] have the tools that they need to be successful in life.

- What comes to mind when you consider what you receive from your students?
- What do you receive from being a teacher?

Chapter Fourteen

What Makes Great Teachers Great?

Contrary to popular lore, teachers do not have eyes in the backs of their heads. They do not see everything. None of us do. In fact, humility about limitations in human perception can be helpful. As Goleman writes, "There is a particular paradox when it comes to confronting the ways in which we do not see. . . . The range of what we think and do is limited by what we fail to notice. And because we fail to notice *that* we fail to notice, there is little we can do to change, until we notice, how failing to notice, shapes our thoughts and deeds."[1]

- What comes to mind when you consider how what you notice and what you fail to notice shapes your thoughts and actions?

What you just considered relates to the question that is the focus of this last chapter. It is the most commonly asked question about the research on exemplary teachers: *What is it that makes great teachers great?*

- How would you answer that question?

While we may have a consistent desire for a simple concise answer, *many* things influence a teacher's success. Human behavior is complex and, importantly, does not occur in a vacuum. A person's thoughts and feelings arise in concert with an experience within a cultural environment. Humans are a social species. We affect and are influenced by one another. That being said, one important thing that helps great teachers be great is their perspicacity. The students, parents and caregivers, colleagues, and all others with whom the teacher comes into contact are affected by the teacher's perspicacity, as well.

Perspicacity refers to the "acuteness of perception, discernment, or understanding."[2] Perspicacity is also defined as "intelligence manifested by being astute" and the "capacity to assess situations or circumstances shrewdly and to draw sound conclusions."[3]

- In what ways can a teacher's perspicacity influence educational outcomes?

WHERE DO OUR ACTIONS COME FROM?

According to the Massachusetts Institute of Technology's C. Otto Scharmer, the "quality of how we pay attention is a largely hidden dimension of our everyday social experience."[4] As we move through our day, we typically are "well aware of *what* we do and *how* we do it—that is, the processes we use. But if we were asked where our actions come from, most of us would be unable to provide a clear response."[5]

Inquiry into the origins and nature of what captures our attention and how we make sense of it is relevant in education. As Rachel said, you need to "be able to think on your feet. . . . You have to do it all day, every day." Cuban uses the word *improvisation* to describe much of what occurs when teaching (see Chapter 12).[6] When improvising and thinking on their feet, teachers scan their environments and access their conscious and unconscious memories. They recognize what to avoid and consider what they could do next.[7]

Although educators' approaches when teaching may be similar, their experience is highly personal. The nature of each teacher's scanning, the memories retrieved, and the perceived options for action, along with quality of the teachers' perspicacity, are all individualized processes. As Palmer suggests, teachers teach who they are.[8]

CULTIVATING PERSPICACITY

It can be helpful to remember that people are not fixed beings. A growing body of research demonstrates that it is possible to shift habitual noticing, broaden interpretations, and expand understanding.[9] The following are vehicles for developing and honing perspicacity:

Self-awareness—Knowing where attention is focused, along with an understanding of one's corresponding thoughts, feelings, and beliefs and the ways these inform and shape personal experience in the moment and over time.

Humility—A deep appreciation that all has not been seen and all is not already known. Tangney identifies six key elements of humility:

1. the accurate assessment of one's abilities and achievement.
2. the ability to acknowledge one's mistakes, imperfections, gaps in knowledge, and limitations.
3. the openness to new ideas, contradictory information, and advice.
4. the keeping of one's abilities and accomplishments . . . in perspective.
5. the relatively low self-focus . . . while recognizing that one is but one part of the larger universe.
6. the appreciation of the value of all things, as well as the many different ways that people and things can contribute to our world.[10]

Curiosity—An energized pursuit of that which is not yet known or well understood; a wanting to know more (e.g., the 3 *I*s)

- *Intellectual curiosity*—A wanting to know information (e.g., content, pedagogy, student development theory, cause-and-effect systems, learning and brain research findings)
- *Interpersonal curiosity*—Seeking connections with and understanding of others (e.g., students, parents and caregivers, colleagues) as well as interest in understanding the larger relational and cultural dynamic operating in all aspects of schools and schooling processes.
- *Intrapersonal curiosity*—A desire to understand how one's thoughts, feelings, and beliefs have come to play a role in what is happening as well as how the self brought to teaching is influencing other individuals, groups, the overall classroom dynamic, teaching and learning processes, and educational outcomes.

Mindful awareness—An understanding of the placement of focused attention; "paying attention to what [we] think and feel without being carried away by those inner stirrings. This observing awareness creates a platform within the mind from which [people] can weigh [their] thoughts, feelings, and impulses before acting on them. And that moment of pausing, gives [people] a crucial degree of freedom that allows [people] to manage [their] emotions and impulses rather than simply be controlled by them."[11]

Compassion—A recognition of hardship and suffering coupled with the desire to take action to help in some way. This refers to compassion for others and also for oneself, as in self-compassion.

Meaning and purpose—A clear awareness and appreciation of the value of one's actions.

Agility skills—According to David, emotional agility allows us to productively negotiate life's inevitable challenges:

> Emotional agility is a process that enables us to navigate life's twists and turns with self-acceptance, clear-sightedness, and an open mind. The process isn't about ignoring difficult emotions and thoughts. It's about holding those emotions and thoughts loosely, facing them courageously and compassionately, and then moving past them to ignite change in your life. . . . [Emotionally agile people] know how to gain critical insight about situations and interactions from their feelings, and use this knowledge to adapt, align their values and actions, and make changes to bring the best of themselves forward.[12]

Hope—According to Lopez, hope is a "belief that the future will be better than the present, along with a belief that you have the power to make it so."[13] This involves an understanding of how to nurture hope in action (meaningful goals, agency thinking, pathway thinking) in oneself and others.

Appreciation skills—These include thankfulness, gratitude, savoring, and the habitual noticing of what is working well in addition to seeing what is not working well.

Positivity—An orientation to actively seek, value, and remember the positive in a person or situation and the willingness to share the positive with others.

Perseverance—A grounded desire and capacity to continue through hardship. This focused use of valuable energy is supported through help and guidance from others.

Self-management—Knowing oneself, along with the prudent use of a variety of well-considered options for situational response (especially when faced with a challenge), such that there is a positive outcome for oneself and others.

Strengths awareness—An understanding and appreciation of one's personal strengths and how to best use them, the capacity to easily spot the strengths in others, and the ability to help others identify and make good use of their strengths.

- What might be some other variables that can support a shift in habitual noticing and understanding?

A friend who is also a teacher suggested I create an acronym to make the previous list of ideas easier to remember. Creating an acronym was a little like playing Scrabble. Moving the letters around yielded the acronym (CHAMPS)[2]:

> Curiosity
> Compassion
> Humility
> Hope
> Agility skills
> Appreciation skills
> Meaning and purpose
> Mindful awareness
> Perseverance
> Positivity
> Self-awareness and self-management
> Strengths awareness

- How might experimenting with one or more of these (CHAMPS)[2] concepts and skills shift what you tend to see, think, and feel and, ultimately, how you might act?

WHAT WE ARE PREPARED TO SEE

The application of the skills that make up (CHAMPS)[2] influences where and how people focus their attention and how they make sense of what they have seen. This influence is important because, as Eberhardt describes, we see the world according to what we are prepared to see: "Our brains are constantly being bombarded with stimuli. And just as we categorize to impose order and coherence on that chaos, we use selective attention to tune in to what seems most salient. Science has shown that people don't attend willy-nilly to things. We choose what to pay attention to based on the ideas that we already have in our heads."[14] The limited information gleaned in a moment, along with the interpretation of that information, work together to help create a person's sense of what is happening and why. Importantly, it also affects a teacher's sense of what is possible.

- How might a teacher benefit, personally and professionally, from experimenting with different approaches to develop and hone perspicacity?
- In what ways could cultivating (CHAMPS)² support a teacher's ability to avoid burnout, find fuel, and cultivate success?

Appendixes

In Appendixes A–F, there is additional information related to educator well-being and materials and exercises to support your teaching practices. The offerings are intentionally varied because different educators have different needs and interests. As you explore this section, I hope you will find some information that helps you avoid burnout, find fuel, and continue to cultivate success.

This section includes:

Appendix A: The Tale of the Stonecutters
Appendix B: Knowing My Students
Appendix C: Staff Directory of Support
Appendix D: Standpoint Exploration
Appendix E: Exploring Hope
Appendix F: Free Resources and Additional Materials

1. Experiences of Teachers of Color
2. Inattentional Blindness, Change Blindness, and Selective Attention
3. Bias, Implicit Cognition, and Educational Equity
4. Faculty Protocols and Activities
5. Mindfulness, Compassion, and Gratitude
6. Additional Information

Appendix A

The Tale of the Stonecutters

Please read the following adaptation of an old story, and see what connections you can make between it and the ideas in this book.

Once upon a time, a hot and weary traveler began to hear lots of extremely loud banging from just ahead along his path. Walking slowly, the traveler came upon a large clearing surrounded by enormous stones.

Moving farther, the traveler spied the source of the sound. It was hammers hitting chisels hitting stone. Four men clearly glistening with sweat were creating the loud racket in four different areas of the huge clearing.

After watching the first worker toil away at his task, the traveler walked closer and asked, "What are you doing?"

The first worker looked up and said, "See these rocks?" pointing to the huge nearby stones. "I need to get them cut. This section needs to be done by the end of this week. It's a big job, and I'm hot, tired, and busy, so please move along."

The traveler took the first stonecutter's suggestion and moved toward the second worker. After watching the rhythmic clanging for a few moments, the traveler asked, "What are you doing?"

The second worker said, "I am cutting these stones. It is a dangerous job that takes much training and experience. I have become known as one of the best stonecutters in our community. If you'll excuse me, I need to get back to my work."

The traveler thanked the second worker and then walked to where the third was located. Again, the traveler watched for a little while and then asked, "What are you doing?"

The third worker paused for a moment and replied, "I am providing for my family. Doing this work makes it possible for my children to have warm clothes, plenty of food, and a solid roof over their heads." Then, with a nod and a smile, he went back to work.

Next, the traveler walked toward the last worker's location. He watched for a short time and then asked, "What are you doing?"

The fourth stonecutter stopped working, slowly raised his eyes, and said with a satisfied smile, "I am building a cathedral."

Appendix B

Knowing My Students

Part I: The following chart provides a structure for you to identify each of your student's (1) interests and hobbies; (2) academic strengths (subjects, skills); (3) personal strengths (qualities, attributes); and (4) what you connect with. Completing the exercise can solidify what you already know about your class as individuals. It also may help identify opportunities to get to know students better.

Student Name	Interests & Hobbies	Academic Strengths	Personal Strengths	What I Connect With

Part II: While filling in the blocks for each student, you may have found that ideas came more easily for some students than others. I invite you to consider why it might be easier to fill in some students' blocks and not others? Who are the students? What is the nature of the teacher-student relationship? What difference might that make? What are some things you might do as a result of completing this exercise?

- Consider connections you can make between this exercise and the information shared in Chapters 4 and 5.
- What might happen if your whole staff adapted this exercise and applied it to all the students in the school?

For example, an administrator could provide school rosters and ask the staff to use three different-colored markers to identify the quality of the student-adult relationship (e.g., color 1 = the adult recognizes the student's name, color 2 = the adult knows the student's academic standing, and color 3 = the adult and student have a personal connection). For additional approaches to gathering and sharing this student information, please see the last two Edutopia links listed under Additional Information in Appendix F.

- Why might it be important to know this information?
- Once known, how might the information be productively considered?
- What connections can you make between this exercise and the ideas in Chapters 9 and 10?

Appendix C

Staff Directory of Support

- How well do you know your colleagues?
- How do you know who to go to for support?
- How do you currently find out about a staff member's area of expertise?

The following chart provides an opportunity to nurture the adult relationships in your school.

Staff Directory of Support

Staff Member Name	Interests and Hobbies	Favorite Subjects to Teach	Preferred Teaching Methods	Materials and Expertise to Share

- What are some different approaches that could be used to gather and share this information?
- Given the information found in Chapters 9 and 10, in what ways might knowing more about one another support educational outcomes?

Appendix D

Standpoint Exploration

- Why don't people always notice the same things? And in those situations where the same things do stand out to people, why can interpretations differ?

Standpoint theory may provide some of the answers. According to Smith and Lee, what each person knows throughout life arises from experiences that occur in a particular time, in a particular place, for a particular person. Where people are positioned in a society affects what is learned, how it is learned, and why it is learned.[1] This is the essence of standpoint theory. Each person's standpoint influences what is made conspicuous in a situation and how that information is interpreted. It also affects what a person misses and ignores.[2]

- Where are you positioned in society?
- In what ways throughout your life has your societal position influenced what you have learned, how you have learned, and why you have learned? How might it affect the relationships you create with others?

Each person's construction of understanding is informed by life experiences. Smith highlights different embedded societal privileges that profoundly affect life experience and a person's standpoint development.[3] An example of this are those privileges that favor upper-class white males in contrast to the privileges offered to women, most notably women of color.[4]

Smith asserts that a person's standpoint is inescapable; it permeates all aspects of a person's life.[5] Lee agrees by suggesting that each educator's standpoint creates a subjectivity that influences all aspects of an educator's teaching practice. Lee reminds educators to not try to deny the existence of their subjectivity; instead, she highlights the value of engaging in thoughtful processes that question it, investigate it, and transform it.[6]

- In what ways does your standpoint influence your teaching practice?
- How do these ideas relate to the information in Chapter 14?

If people have similarities (e.g., socioeconomic status, ethnicity, schooling, personality, age, gender, social class, etc.), they may be more likely to notice some of the same situational variables and interpret them in a similar way. However, with a more diverse group, different situational variables may be noticed. In *The Power of Diversity*, Geraldine Richmond explains how, in scientific research settings, "examples abound that show how a diverse team can identify and address issues a like-minded and a look-alike team might miss."[7]

- How diverse is your school staff (e.g., socioeconomic status, ethnicity, schooling, personality, age, gender, social class, etc.)? In what ways does your school staff's level of diversity influence what is noticed and how that information is understood?
- What can be challenging about conversations when different perspectives are heard?
- What are some benefits of conversations when diverse views are valued?
- How might the information in Chapters 2, 9, and 10 connect with your ideas concerning standpoint theory?

Appendix E

Exploring Hope

As mentioned in Chapter 9, Lopez describes hope-in-action as having three parts—meaningful goals, agency thinking, and pathway thinking—that synergistically act as a powerful feedback loop for human behavior. When at least one of the three weakens, we experience a loss of hope.[1] As you read on, consider how each may relate to you:

Meaningful goals arise from consideration of questions related to a desired future self (e.g., Who do I want to be? What do I most want to do? Where do I want to go?). Meaningful goals act as an organizing force. They help pull the person forward.[2]

Agency thinking is a type of cause-and-effect-based belief in a personal ability to shape one's own life; to motivate oneself; and to persist when pursuing long-term, personally meaningful goals. It involves understanding personal talents, skills, and strengths, as well as appreciating outside supports ready to be tapped in service of starting and persisting toward meaningful goals.[3]

Pathway thinking refers to an awareness of multiple routes toward a desired outcome, the evaluation of options, the monitoring of progress, the expectation of possible hardship and challenge, and an open and curious stance that enables the uncovering and consideration of additional options forward.

- How might your processes of reflection cultivate your meaningful goals, agency thinking, and pathway thinking?

- In what ways do you support your students' cultivation of meaningful goals, agency thinking, and pathway thinking, thereby supporting their experiences of hope?

Lopez views hope as the work of the head (thoughts) and the heart (emotions). Thoughts and feelings are intertwined brain processes. The strong desire inherent in a person's meaningful goals causes an inspiring emotional response. This compelling emotional tenor supports resilience and persistence during goal pursuit. A person's cognitive grounding—involving the consideration of meaningful goals, pathway thinking, and agency thinking—supports the thoughtful negotiation of emotional content. This in turn causes a synergistic movement toward potent, highly desired future possibilities.[4]

A person's experience of hope is fostered in each moment through making deliberate choices. Lopez explains, "It happens when we use our thoughts and feelings to temper our aversion to loss and actively pursue what is possible. When we choose hope, we define what matters most to us."[5] According to Scioli and Biller, we see this "whenever disaster strikes. . . . We all look for hope. . . . We look for hope to sustain us, whenever and wherever we can."[6]

- When has hope supported your resilience through hardship?

Humans tell themselves powerful stories about their past (reliving) and future (preliving). Past memories create a point from which to compare and contrast a potential future. This personal narrative affects a person's sense of hope concerning what is possible.[7]

Due to neural plasticity, a person's internal story line can change over time and with some degree of disconfirming experiences. The neural networks that anticipate experience and cause perception prioritization can shift, affecting the cultivation of hope.[8] In addition, research suggests that hope can also be nurtured through learning about the positive stories of others.[9]

- In what ways does your internal dialogue concerning what is happening and what is possible inform your experience of hope?
- What connections can you make between your processes of reflection and your internal story line?
- Think about a story you heard or a movie you watched that fostered a sense of hope in you. What was it that captured your attention? How did it influence your thoughts, feelings, and experience of hope?

Frequent policy, program, and curriculum changes can overwhelm teachers, especially if they have little control or influence over changes that directly affect their daily lives.[10] In addition, too much change enacted too rapidly inhibits thoughtful, accurate appraisals of what is occurring, which in turn informs and determines the quality of decision-making.[11]

When people lose their ability to see a better future than the present or they lose their belief that they have what it takes to create that positive vision, they lose hope. In hope's absence, intelligence remains dormant, an underutilized resource. When in a low hope state, people have reduced access to the best of what they know. A loss of hope negatively influences a person's emotional state and thinking processes.[12]

Hope's motivational energy allows for greater use of a person's cognitive abilities. A person's intelligence and hope reinforce each other to positively spur creativity and productivity.[13] Because hope can act as a contagion, a teacher's experience of hope can spread to others (colleagues, administrators, students, parents), thereby affecting their levels of hope.[14]

- Have you ever seen hope or a loss of hope spread between people? What contributed to that experience?
- Have you ever experienced a loss of hope? If so, how did it influence your thinking and feeling?

Sometimes, it can be difficult to see a way out of a challenging situation. As mentioned previously, when the exemplary educators face challenges, they readily seek help from a variety of sources (e.g., school-based programs, administrators, web supports, prior professional learning). They also mine their own past teaching experiences via reflection. For most of the teachers, another major source of support lies in their positive relationships with colleagues. The teachers gain valuable insight from listening with openness and curiosity to their colleagues' perspectives.

We each have a limited system of perception. None of us sees all. However, we each have an opportunity to render our naturally incomplete perception more complete. Because we are a social species, we are hardwired to value interactions with other people with whom we have close ties. Sharing with others can lighten our load and broaden our view.

According to Albert Schweitzer, it is helpful to remember that "at times, our own light goes out and is rekindled by a spark from another person. Each of us has cause to think with deep gratitude of those who have lighted the flame within us."[15]

- Have you ever felt mired in a situation, unable to see a path forward, and then, through sharing the challenge with others, you gained a new perspective? Who was involved? What was the situation? What helped? How were you ultimately able to see things differently?

High-hope people tend to spread hope to others with whom they interact. Recent research suggests hope affects a person's success in school, work, and life. Hope leads to increased academic performance and enhanced workplace outcomes. High-hope students and workers have lower absenteeism and more productivity. Hopeful people tend to have a higher pain tolerance and greater longevity and make better health decisions. According to Lopez, hope-in-action elevates, energizes, and positively affects daily behavior choices.[16] It is vital to the creation of a meaningful life.[17]

- Have you ever felt greater hope after speaking with someone? What were some things that the person said or did that bolstered your sense of hope?
- Consider what you have learned in this book about exemplary educators and hope-in-action. What are some ways the exemplary teachers foster hope in themselves and others?
- How do you nurture hope in others?
- How do you nurture hope in yourself?

To clarify, this understanding of hope differs from what the word *hope* means in the sentences *I hope you have a nice day* or *I hope it doesn't rain tomorrow*. In those examples, the word *hope* is more akin to wishing.[18] This conception of hope also differs from simple optimism. Based in part on temperament, optimism is the general sense that things will turn out positively. Sometimes referred to as positive expectation bias, it has health and happiness benefits. However, when hardships occur, optimists can often struggle and get frustrated. Conversely, hardship energizes high-hope individuals. Hopeful people seek meaning and purpose within the challenge and persevere with dignity. They not only believe that the future will be better than the present, but they also know that they can work to make it so.[19]

- Think about a time when you felt really hopeful as an educator. In what ways might your meaningful goals, pathway thinking, and agency thinking have affected and informed that experience?

Appendix F

Free Resources and Additional Materials

1. EXPERIENCES OF TEACHERS OF COLOR

Through our eyes: Perspectives and reflections from black teachers. https://edtrust.org/wp-content/uploads/2014/09/ThroughOurEyes.pdf

The experiences of teachers of color, Harvard University, Usable knowledge. https://www.gse.harvard.edu/news/uk/18/06/experiences-teachers-color

The research handbook on teachers of color (Gist & Bristol, in press). https://uh.edu/education/research-convening/

2. INATTENTIONAL BLINDNESS, CHANGE BLINDNESS, AND SELECTIVE ATTENTION

Inattentional blindness—Magic Singh—BBC. https://www.youtube.com/watch?v=b7LuvAM6XLg

Inattentional blindness—Double dutch—Brain Games—National Geographic. https://www.youtube.com/watch?v=TSsuwZvom3g

Change blindness, speed of changes, spatial awareness—Brain Games—National Geographic. https://www.youtube.com/watch?v=_FoghxotdYU

Selective attention and inattentional blindness—Whodunnit?—Transport for London. https://www.youtube.com/watch?v=ubNF9QNEQLA

Divided attention, selective attention, inattentional blindness, change blindness—Khan Academy. https://www.youtube.com/watch?v=s4JBqLoY3tY

3. BIAS, IMPLICIT COGNITION, AND EDUCATIONAL EQUITY

Project Implicit, Harvard University. https://implicit.harvard.edu/implicit/

Awareness of implicit biases, Yale University Poorvu Center for Teaching and Learning. https://poorvucenter.yale.edu/ImplicitBiasAwareness

The Ohio State University Kirwan Institute for the Study of Race and Ethnicity. http://kirwaninstitute.osu.edu/?s=implicit+bias

Equity resources, Collaborating States Initiative (CSI). https://casel.org/csi-resources-equity/

National Equity Project. https://nationalequityproject.org

Designing for equity, Next Generation Learning Challenges. https://www.nextgenlearning.org/challenges/designing-for-equity. https://www.nextgenlearning.org/equity-toolkit

Zaretta Hammond, Culturally Responsive Teaching and the Brain. https://www.youtube.com/watch?v=9nMK1nepwvk

4. FACULTY PROTOCOLS AND ACTIVITIES

National school reform faculty protocols and activities (as cited by Fiarman, 2017, p. 1). https://nsrfharmony.org/protocols/

Data Wise: Educators collaborating so all students thrive (as cited by Fiarman, 2017, p. 1). https://datawise.gse.harvard.edu

Meeting Wise: Making the most of collaborative time (as cited by Fiarman, 2017, p. 1). https://www.hepg.org/hep-home/books/meeting-wise

Benefits of active constructive responding, Institute of Positive Education, Geelong Grammar. https://www.ggs.vic.edu.au/Blog-Posts/the-benefits-of-active-constructive-responding

Capitalizing on positive events, Greater Good in Action, University of California, Berkeley. https://ggia.berkeley.edu/practice/capitalizing_on_positive_events

Active listening, Greater Good in Action, University of California, Berkeley. https://ggia.berkeley.edu/practice/active_listening

Three signature practices, CASEL Guide to Schoolwide SEL, https://schoolguide.casel.org/resource/three-signature-sel-practices-for-adult-learning/

Adult school community, CASEL, Collaborating States Initiative (CSI) https://casel.org/csi-resources-professional-learning/

Adult SEL, CASEL, SEL Implementation Tools and Resources. https://casel.org/resources-support/

5. MINDFULNESS, COMPASSION, AND GRATITUDE

Mindful Awareness Research Center (MARC) at the University of California, Los Angeles. https://www.uclahealth.org/marc/mindful-meditations

Mindfulness in schools. https://www.mindfulschools.org/about-mindfulness/research-on-mindfulness/

Awe walk, Greater Good in Action, University of California, Berkeley. https://ggia.berkeley.edu/practice/awe_walk

Compassion training, Center for Healthy Minds, University of Wisconsin, Madison. https://centerhealthyminds.org/join-the-movement/compassion-training

Compassion and high expectations. https://www.edutopia.org/article/necessity-having-high-expectations

Self-Compassion exercises—Kristin Neff, Ph.D., University of Texas, Austin. https://self-compassion.org/category/exercises/

Gratitude curricula, The Greater Good in Education (GGIE), University of California, Berkeley. https://ggsc.berkeley.edu/who_we_serve/educators/educator_resources/gratitude_curricula

Gratitude letter, Greater Good in Action, University of California, Berkeley. https://ggia.berkeley.edu/practice/gratitude_letter

Three good things, Greater Good in Action, University of California, Berkeley. https://ggia.berkeley.edu/practice/three-good-things

Practice finding silver linings, Greater Good in Action, University of California, Berkeley. https://ggia.berkeley.edu/practice/finding_silver_linings

Savoring walk, Greater Good in Action, University of California, Berkeley. https://ggia.berkeley.edu/practice/savoring_walk

6. ADDITIONAL INFORMATION

Expressive writing, Greater Good in Action, University of California, Berkeley. https://ggia.berkeley.edu/practice/expressive_writing

Wellbeing toolkit, Center for Healthy Minds at the University of Wisconsin, Madison. https://hminnovations.org/hmi/resources/your-well-being-toolkit

Open-source ideas, tools, and strategies, Next Generation Learning Challenges. https://www.nextgenlearning.org/resources?challenge=0&topics=&media=0&audiences=0&page=1

Videos & resources, National Commission on Social, Emotional, and Academic Development. http://nationathope.org

Resources, The Greater Good in Education (GGIE), University of California, Berkeley. https://ggsc.berkeley.edu/who_we_serve/educators/educator_resources/ggie

The CASEL Guide to Schoolwide Social and Emotional Learning. https://schoolguide.casel.org

IPEN Learning Library, International Positive Education Network. http://ipen-network.com/learningcontents

Short video series, International Positive Psychology Association. http://www.ippanetwork.org/ppvideos/

Directory of free practices, Greater Good in Action, University of California, Berkeley. https://ggia.berkeley.edu

Three funny things, Greater Good in Action, University of California, Berkeley. https://ggia.berkeley.edu/practice/three_funny_things

Gaining perspective on negative events, Greater Good in Action, University of California. https://ggia.berkeley.edu/practice/gaining_perspective_on_negative_events

Use your strengths, Greater Good in Action, University of California, Berkeley. https://ggia.berkeley.edu/practice/use_your_strengths

Free strengths identification, VIA Science of Strengths, Practice of Wellbeing. https://www.viacharacter.org/www/

About using the Via Survey of Character Strengths, Michelle McQuaid, Ph.D. https://www.michellemcquaid.com/via-survey-character-strengths/

Making sure each student is known, Edutopia. https://www.edutopia.org/video/making-sure-each-child-known

Knowing every student through index card rosters, Edutopia. https://www.edutopia.org/video/knowing-every-child-through-index-card-rosters

Notes

INTRODUCTION

1. Herman, K. C., Hickmon-Rosa, J., & Reinke, W. M. (2018), Empirically derived profiles of teacher stress, burnout, self-efficacy, and coping and associated student outcomes, *Journal of Positive Behavior Interventions*, *20*(2), 90–100.
2. Palmer, P. (2007), *Courage to teach* (San Francisco: Jossey-Bass), 69.
3. Fisher, B. (1998), *Joyful learning in kindergarten* (Portsmouth, NH: Heinemann).
4. Levy, S. (1996), *Starting from scratch: One classroom builds its own curriculum* (Portsmouth, NH: Heinemann).
5. Balonon-Rosen, P. (2016, January 7), Massachusetts education again ranks no. 1 nationally, Learning Lab, retrieved from http://learninglab.legacy.wbur.org/2016/01/07/massachusetts-education-again-ranks-no-1-nationally/; Massachusetts earns a B-plus on state report card, ranks first in nation (2018, January), *Education Week*, retrieved fromhttps://www.edweek.org/ew/collections/quality-counts-2018-state-grades/highlight-reports/2018/01/17/massachusetts.html
6. Massachusetts Department of Education (2018), Educator evaluation data 2015–2016, retrieved fromhttp://profiles.doe.mass.edu/statereport/educatorevaluationperformance.aspx
7. Massachusetts Model System for Educator Evaluation (2015, December), *Part III: Guide to rubrics and model rubrics for superintendent, administrator, and teacher* (Malden: Massachusetts Department of Elementary and Secondary Education), 10.
8. Massachusetts Department of Education (2018), Educator evaluation, retrieved fromhttp://www.doe.mass.edu/edeval/resources/rubrics/, 1.
9. Jenko, M. (2014, March 13), EBP lecture for module 3: Qualitative research designs, descriptive statistics, retrieved fromhttps://www.youtube.com/watch?v=ooNQmha-3Bw
10. Creswell, J. W. (2008), *Educational research: Planning, conducting, and evaluating quantitative and qualitative research* (Upper Saddle River, NJ: Pearson).
11. Merriam, S. B. (2009), *Qualitative research: A guide to design and implementation* (San Francisco: Jossey-Bass).
12. Guest, G., Bunce, A., & Johnson, L. (2006), How many interviews are enough? An experiment with data saturation and variability, *Field Methods*, *18*(1), 59–82.

HOW TEACHERS SEE THEIR WORK

1. Walker, T. (2018, May 11), How many teachers are highly stressed? Maybe more people than your think, *NEA Today*, 18, retrieved fromhttp://neatoday.org/2018/05/11/study-high-teacher-stress-levels/

2. Jordan, J. V. (2017, October), Relational-Cultural Theory: The power of connection to transform our lives, *Journal of Humanistic Counseling*, 56(3), 234.

3. Lieberman, M. D. (2014), *Social: Why our brains are wired to connect* (New York: Crown), 132; Schwartz, H. L. (2019), *Connected teaching: Relationship, power, and mattering in higher education* (Sterling, VA: Stylus).

4. Wrzesniewski, A., Dutton, J., & Debebe, G. (2003), Interpersonal sensemaking and the meaning of work, *Research in Organizational Behavior*, 25, 93–135.

5. Wrzesniewski, Dutton, & Debebe, Interpersonal sensemaking; Berg, J. M., Dutton, J. E., & Wrzesniewski, A. (2013), Job crafting and meaningful work, in *Purpose and meaning in the workplace*, B. J. Dik., Z. S. Byrne, & M. F. Steger (Eds.) (Washington, DC: American Psychological Association), 83.

6. Wrzesniewski, Dutton, & Debebe, Interpersonal sensemaking.

7. Wrzesniewski, A. (2014, November 10), Job crafting: How individuals revision work, re: Work with Google [video file], retrieved from https://www.youtube.com/watch?v=C_igfnctYjA

8. Wrzesniewski, A., & Dutton, J. E. (2001), Crafting a job: Revisioning employees as active crafters of their work, *Academy of Management Review*, 26, 179–201; Wrzesniewski, Dutton, & Debebe, Interpersonal sensemaking.

9. Dik, Byrne, & Steger, *Purpose and meaning*; Langer, E. J. (2014), *Mindfulness* (Reading, MA: Addison-Wesley); Neault, R. A. (Ed.) (2011), *Thoughts on theories* [Special issue], *Journal of Employment Counseling*, 48(4).

10. Grant, A. (2018, January 11), Who we are: Collaborators, *Ethical Systems*, 1, retrieved from https://www.ethicalsystems.org/content/who-we-are

1. TEACHER POWER

1. McGrath, H., & Noble, T. (2010), Supporting positive pupil relationships: Research to practice. *Education & Child Psychology*, 27(1), 79–90.

2. Sizer, T. R., & Faust Sizer, N. (1999), *The students are watching: Schools and the moral contract* (Boston: Beacon Press).

3. Senge, P., Cambron-McCabe, N., Lucas, T., Smith, B., Dutton, J., & Kleiner, A. (2012), *Schools that learn: A fifth discipline fieldbook for educators, parents, and everyone who cares about education* (New York: Random House).

4. Singer, T., & Bolz, M. (Eds.) (2014), *Compassion: Bridging practice and science* (Munich: Max Planck Society), 6.

Note: Item 13 (Burnout n.d., Lexico) retrieved fromhttps://en.oxforddictionaries.com/definition/burnout

5. Siegel, D. J. (2010), *Mindsight: The new science of personal transformation* (New York: Random House); Munoz, L. M. P. (2013, June 24), Feeling others' pain: Transforming empathy into compassion, Cognitive Neuroscience Society, retrieved fromhttps://www.cogneurosociety.org/empathy_pain/

6. Seppala, E. (2019, November 7), Four ways to calm your mind in stressful times, *Greater Good Magazine*, retrieved fromhttps://greatergood.berkeley.edu/article/item/four_ways_to_calm_your_mind_in_stressful_times

7. Mahoney, H. M. (2017, August 2), The other side of empathy, Medium, retrieved from https://medium.com/stanford-d-school/the-other-side-of-empathy-6c1512aa2963

8. Munoz, Feeling others' pain.

2. THE GIFT OF PROVIDING A FRESH START

1. Eberhardt, J. L. (2019), *Biased: Uncovering the hidden prejudice that shapes what we see, think, and do* (New York: Viking); Pielmeier, M., Huber, S., & Seidel, T. (2018), Is teacher judgment accuracy of students' characteristics beneficial for verbal teacher-student interactions in the classroom? *Teaching and Teacher Education*, 76(11), 255–266; Senge, P., Cambron-McCabe, N., Lucas, T., Smith, B., Dutton, J., & Kleiner, A. (2012), *Schools that learn: A fifth discipline fieldbook for educators, parents, and everyone who cares about education* (New York: Random House).

2. Eagleman, D. (2015), *The brain: The story of you* (New York: Penguin Random House); Goleman, D. (2006), *Social intelligence: The new science of human relationships* (New York: Bantam Dell); McGonigal, K. (2012), *The neuroscience of change* (Louisville, CO: Sounds True).

3. Olson, K. (2014), *The invisible classroom: Relationships, neuroscience, and mindfulness in school* (New York: W. W. Norton).

4. Olson, *Invisible classroom*.

5. McNerney, S. (2011), Confirmation bias and art, *Scientific American*, retrieved fromhttp://blogs.scientificamerican.com/guest-blog/confirmation-bias-and-art/; Nickerson, R. S. (1998), Confirmation bias: A ubiquitous phenomenon in many guises. *Review of General Psychology*, 2(2), 175–220.

6. Eberhardt, *Biased*, 33.

7. Frost, P., Casey, B., Griffin, K., Raymundo, L., Farrell, C., & Carrigan, R. (2015), The influence of confirmation bias on memory and source monitoring, *Journal of General Psychology*, 142(4), 238–252.

8. Chen, M., & Bargh, J. A. (1997), Nonconscious behavioral confirmation processes: The self-fulfilling consequences of automatic stereotype activation, *Journal of Experimental Social Psychology*, 33, 541–560; Eagleman, *The brain*; Staats, C., & Contractor, D. (2014), *Race and discipline in Ohio schools: What the data say* (Columbus: Kirwan Institute for the Study of Race and Ethnicity at Ohio State University).

9. Deal, T. E., & Kennedy, A. A. (1983, February), Culture and school performance, *Educational Leadership*, 40(5), 14.

10. Hammond, Z. (2015), *Culturally responsive teaching and the brain* (Thousand Oaks, CA: Sage); Hollins, E. R. (2008), *Culture in school learning: Revealing the deep meaning* (New York: Routledge); Staats & Contractor, *Race and discipline*.

11. Gay, G. (2010), *Culturally responsive teaching* (New York: Teachers College).

12. Gay, *Culturally responsive teaching*.

13. Hollins, *Culture in school learning*; Mason, B. A., Gunersel, A. B., & Ney, E. A. (2014), Cultural and ethnic bias in teacher ratings of behavior: A criterion-focused review, *Psychology in the Schools*, *51*(10), 1017–1030; Staats & Contractor, *Race and discipline*.

3. MEANING AND PURPOSE

1. Berg, J. M., Dutton, J. E., & Wrzesniewski, A. (2013), Job crafting and meaningful work, in *Purpose and Meaning in the Workplace*, B. J. Dik., Z. S. Byrne, & M. F. Steger (Eds.) (Washington, DC: American Psychological Association), 80–10; Langer, E. J. (2014), *Mindfulness* (Reading, MA: Addison-Wesley); Wrzesniewski, A., & Dutton, J. E. (2001), Crafting a job: Revisioning employees as active crafters of their work, *Academy of Management Review*, *26*, 179–201; Wrzesniewski, A., Dutton, J. E., & Debebe, G. (2003), Interpersonal sensemaking and the meaning of work, *Research in Organizational Behavior*, *25*, 93–135; Wrzesniewski, A., McCauley, C., Rozin, P., & Schwartz, B. (1997), Jobs, careers, and callings: People's relations to their work, *Journal of Research in Personality*, *31*, 21–33.

2. Grant, A. (2018, November 12), Who we are: Collaborators, Ethical Systems, retrieved fromhttps://www.ethicalsystems.org/content/who-we-are

3. Santoro, D. A. (2018), *Demoralized: Why teachers leave the profession they love and how they can stay* (Cambridge, MA: Harvard Education Press).

4. Santoro, D. A. (2018), Is it burnout? Or demoralization? *Educational Leadership*, *75*(6), 12.

5. Santoro, Is it burnout? 12.

6. Santoro, D. (2011), Good teaching in difficult times: Demoralization in the pursuit of good work, *American Journal of Education*, *118*(1), 14.

7. Santoro, Good teaching, 18.

8. Santoro, *Demoralized*.

9. Santoro, Is it burnout? 15.

4. KNOWING STUDENTS WELL

1. Capp, M. J. (2017), The effectiveness of universal design for learning: A meta-analysis of literature between 2013 and 2016, *International Journal of Inclusive Education*, *21*(8), 791–793.

2. Jupp, J. C. (2013), *Becoming teachers of inner-city students: Life histories and teacher stories of committed white teachers* (Rotterdam, Netherlands: Sense).

3. Pope, R. L., Reynolds, A. L., & Mueller, J. A. (2014), *Creating multicultural change on campus* (San Francisco: Jossey-Bass).

4. Eberhardt, J. L. (2019), *Biased: Uncovering the hidden prejudice that shapes what we see, think, and do* (New York: Viking), 48.

5. Phillips, D. K., & Carr, K. (2014), *Becoming a teacher through action research: Process, context, and self-study* (New York: Taylor & Francis); Staats, C. (2015), Understanding implicit bias: What educators should know, *American Educator*, retrieved fromhttp://www.aft.org/ae/winter2015-2016/staats

6. Gay, G. (2010), *Culturally responsive teaching* (New York: Teachers College).

7. Gaitan, C. D. (2006), *Building culturally responsive classrooms* (Thousand Oaks, CA: Sage).

8. Berardo, K., & Deardorff, D. (2012), *Building cultural competence: Innovative activities and models* (Sterling, VA: Stylus); Staats, Understanding implicit bias; Strouse, J. H. (2001), *Exploring socio-cultural themes in education* (Columbus, OH: Prentice-Hall).

9. Hammond, Z. (2015), *Culturally responsive teaching and the brain* (Thousand Oaks, CA: Sage), 15.

10. Brookfield, S. D. (2009), *The skillful teacher: On technique, trust, and responsiveness in the classroom* (San Francisco: Wiley).

5. CULTIVATING POSITIVE RELATIONSHIPS WITH STUDENTS

1. Gregory, M., & Gregory, M. V. (2013), *Teaching excellence in higher education* (New York: Palgrave Macmillan).

2. Bandura, A. (1986), *Social foundations of thought and action: A social cognitive theory* (Englewood Cliffs, NJ: Prentice-Hall); Eagleman, D. (2015), *The brain: The story of you* (New York: Penguin Random House); Surrey, J., & Kramer, G. (2013), Relational mindfulness, in C. K. Germer, R. D. Siegel, & P. R. Fulton (Eds.), *Mindfulness and psychotherapy* (94–111) (New York: Guilford).

3. Schwartz, H. L. (2019), *Connected teaching: Relationship, power, and mattering in higher education* (Sterling, VA: Stylus), 33–34.

4. Walker, M. (2004), How relationships heal, in M. Walker & W. B. Rosen (Eds.), *How connections heal: Stories from relational-cultural therapy* (3–21) (New York: Guilford Press), 34; Schwartz, *Connected teaching*.

5. Gregory & Gregory, *Teaching excellence*.

6. Jacobs, H. H. (2010), *Curriculum 21: Essential education for a changing world* (Alexandria, VA: ASCD), 2.

7. Groccia, J. E. (2018, Summer), What is student engagement? *New Directions for Teaching and Learning*, no. 154, 11–20; Schlechty, P. C. (2001), *Shaking up the schoolhouse: How to support and sustain educational innovation* (San Francisco: Jossey-Bass).

8. Bransford, J. D., Brown, A. L., & Cocking, R. R. (2000), *How people learn* (Washington, DC: National Academy Press); Kober, N. (2015), *Reaching students: What research says about effective instruction in undergraduate science and engineering* (Washington, DC: National Academies Press).

9. Style, E. J. (2014), Curriculum as encounter: Selves and shelves, *English Journal*, *103*(5), 67.

10. Goleman, D., & Senge, P. (2014), *The triple focus: A new approach to education* (Florence, MA: More Than Sound), 14.

11. Kytle, J. (2004), *To want to learn* (New York: Palgrave Macmillan).

12. Freemark, S. (2014, October 16), Studying with quizzes helps make sure the material sticks, Mindshift, retrieved from https://www.kqed.org/mindshift/37752/studying-with-quizzes-helps-make-sure-the-material-sticks

13. Dweck, C. (2000), *Self-theories* (Philadelphia: Taylor & Francis); Dweck, C. S. (2006), *Mindset: The new psychology of success* (New York: Random House).

14. Niemiec, R. M. (2018), *Character strengths interventions: A field guide* (Boston: Hogrefe); Niemiec, R. M., & McGrath, R. E. (2019), *The power of character strengths: Appreciate and ignite your positive personality* (Cincinnati, OH: VIA Institute on Character); Yeager, J. M., Fisher, S. W., & Shearon, D. N. (2011), *Smart strengths: Building character, resilience and relationships in youth* (Putnam Valley, NY: Kravis).

15. Collaborative for Academic, Social, and Emotional Learning (2019), Core SEL competencies, retrieved from https://casel.org/core-competencies/

16. Miller, J. B. (1976), *Toward a new psychology of women* (Boston: Beacon Press); Miller, J. B. (1986), *What do we mean by relationships?* (Work in Progress No. 22) (Wellesley, MA: Stone Center Working Paper Series); Miller, J. B. (2008), How change happens: Controlling images, mutuality, and power, *Women & Therapy, 31*(2–4), 109–127.

17. Gunderson, C., Graff, D., & Craddock, K. (Eds.) (2018), *Transforming community: Stories of connection through the lens of relational-cultural theory* (Duluth, MN: Whole Person).

18. Taxer, J. L., Becker-Kurz, B., & Frenzel, A. C. (2019, February), Do quality teacher–student relationships protect teachers from emotional exhaustion? The mediating role of enjoyment and anger, *Social Psychology of Education, 22*(1), 209.

6. NEGOTIATING DIFFICULT RELATIONSHIPS WITH STUDENTS

1. Collaborative for Academic, Social, and Emotional Learning, (2019), Core SEL competencies, retrieved from https://casel.org/core-competencies/

2. Split, J. L., Koomen, H. M. Y., & Thijs, J. T. (2011), Teacher wellbeing: The importance of teacher–student relationships, *Educational Psychology Review, 23*(4), 457–477.

3. Olson, K. (2014), *The invisible classroom: Relationships, neuroscience, and mindfulness in school* (New York: W. W. Norton).

4. Split, Koomen, & Thijs, Teacher wellbeing.

5. Edwards, C., Edwards, A., Torrens, A., & Beck, A. (2011, October), Confirmation and community: The relationships between teacher confirmation, classroom community, student motivation, and learning, *Online Journal of Communication and Media, 1*(4), 17–43, retrieved from https://www.ojcmt.net/volume-1/issue-4

6. Cullen, M., & Brito Pons, G. (2015), *The mindfulness-based emotional balance workbook* (Oakland, CA: New Harbinger).

7. Milner, R. H. (2011, January/February), Five easy ways to connect with students. *Harvard Education Letter, 27*(1), 1.

8. Jupp, J. C. (2013), *Becoming teachers of inner-city students: Life histories and teacher stories of committed white teachers* (Rotterdam, Netherlands: Sense).

9. Chabris, C. F., & Simons, D. J. (2010), *The invisible gorilla: And other ways our intuitions deceive us* (New York: Random House).

10. Chen, M., & Bargh, J. A. (1997), Nonconscious behavioral confirmation processes: The self-fulfilling consequences of automatic stereotype activation, *Journal of Experimental Social Psychology, 33*, 541–560; Goleman, D. (2013), *Focus: The hidden driver of excellence* (New York: HarperCollins).

11. Achor, S. (2013), *Before happiness: The five hidden keys to achievement* (New York: Random House); Kozak, A. (2009), *Wild chickens and petty tyrants: 108 metaphors for mind-*

fulness (Somerville, MA: Wisdom); Schmidt, R. F. (1986), *Fundamentals of sensory physiology* (New York: Springer).

12. Chabris & Simons, *Invisible gorilla*; Olson, *Invisible classroom*.

13. McNerney, S. (2011), Confirmation bias and art, *Scientific American*, retrieved fromhttp://blogs.scientificamerican.com/guest-blog/confirmation-bias-and-art/; Nickerson, R. S. (1998), Confirmation bias: A ubiquitous phenomenon in many guises, *Review of General Psychology*, 2(2), 175–220.

14. Hanson, R. (2013), *Hardwiring happiness: The new brain science of contentment, calm, and confidence* (New York: Random House); Rozin, P., & Royzman, E. B. (2001), Negativity bias, negativity dominance, and contagion, *Personality and Social Psychology Review*, 5(4), 296–320.

15. Baumeister, R. F., Bratslavsky, E., Finkenauer, C., & Vohs, K. D. (2001), Bad is stronger than good, *Review of General Psychology*, 5(4), 323.

16. Rozin & Royzman, Negativity bias.

17. Baumeister et al., Bad is stronger; Hanson, *Hardwiring happiness*.

18. Appiah, B. (2013, March 14), Selective attention and inattentional blindness: Test your awareness: Whodunnit? EdLab Columbia University [video file], retrieved fromhttps://edlab.tc.columbia.edu/blog/9027-Selective-Attention-and-Inattentional-Blindness

19. Olson, *Invisible classroom*; Simons, D. J., & Chabris, C. F. (1999), Gorillas in our midst: Sustained inattentional blindness for dynamic events, *Perception*, 28, 1059–1074.

20. Simons, D. J. (2000), Attentional capture and inattentional blindness, *Trends in Cognitive Sciences*, 4(4), 147–155.

21. Chabris & Simons, *Invisible gorilla*.

22. Chen & Bargh, Nonconscious behavioral confirmation processes; Staats, C. (2015), Understanding implicit bias: What educators should know, *American Educator*, retrieved fromhttp://www.aft.org/ae/winter2015-2016/staats; Staats, C., & Contractor, D. (2014), *Race and discipline in Ohio schools: What the data say* (Columbus: Kirwan Institute for the Study of Race and Ethnicity at Ohio State University).

23. Chen & Bargh, Nonconscious behavioral confirmation processes; Eagleman, D. (2015), *The brain: The story of you* (New York: Penguin Random House).

24. Surrey, J., & Kramer, G. (2013), Relational mindfulness, in C. K. Germer, R. D. Siegel, & P. R. Fulton (Eds.), *Mindfulness and psychotherapy* (94–111) (New York: Guilford), 106.

25. Fredrickson, B. L. (1998), What good are positive emotions? *Review of General Psychology* [special issue]. *New Directions in Research on Emotion*, 2(3), 300–319; Fredrickson, B. L. (2013), Positive emotions broaden and build, *Advances in Experimental Social Psychology*, 47, 1–53.

26. Singer, T., & Bolz, M. (2014), *Compassion: Bridging practice and science* (Munich, Germany: Max Planck Society).

27. Chabris & Simons, *Invisible gorilla*.

28. Singer & Bolz, *Compassion*.

29. Cullen & Brito Pons, *Mindfulness-based emotional balance*.

30. Kabat-Zinn, J. (2005), *Coming to our senses: Healing ourselves and the world through mindfulness* (New York: Hyperion); Smalley, S. L., & Winston, D. (2010), *Fully present: The science, art, and practice of mindfulness* (Philadelphia: Perseus).

31. Smalley & Winston, *Fully present*, 174.

32. Salzberg, S. (2014), *Real happiness at work* (New York: Workman), 12.

33. Flook, L., Goldberg, S. B., Pinger, L., Bonus, K., & Davidson, R. J. (2013), Mindfulness for teachers: A pilot study to assess effects on stress, burnout and teaching efficacy, *Mind, Brain and Education: The Official Journal of the International Mind, Brain, and Education*

Society, *7*(3), 182–195; Garner, P. W., Bender, S. L., & Fedor, M. (2018), Mindfulness-based SEL programming to increase preservice teachers' mindfulness and emotional competence, *Psychology in the Schools*, *55*(4), 377–390; Hirshberg, M. J., Flook, L., Enright, R. D., & Davidson, R. J. (2020, April), Integrating mindfulness and connection practices into preservice teacher education improves classroom practices, *Learning and Instruction*, *66*, 101298; Jennings, P. A., Frank, J. L., Snowberg, K. E., Coccia, M. A., & Greenberg, M. T. (2013), Improving classroom learning environments by cultivating awareness and resilience in education (CARE): Results of a randomized controlled trial, *School Psychology Quarterly*, *28*(4), 374–390.

34. Schonert-Reichl, K. A., Oberle, E., Lawlor, M. S., Abbott, D., Thomson, K., Oberlander, T. F., & Diamond, A. (2015), Enhancing cognitive and social-emotional development through a simple-to-administer mindfulness-based school program for elementary school children: A randomized controlled trial. *Developmental Psychology*, *51*(1), 52–66; Siblinga, E. M. S., Webb, L., Ghazarian, S. R., & Ellen, J. M. (2016), School-based mindfulness instruction: An RCT, *Pediatrics*, *137*(1), 1–8.

35. Hyland, T. (2011), *Mindfulness and learning* (London: Springer), 105.

36. Goleman, D., & Senge, P. (2014), *The triple focus: A new approach to education* (Florence, MA: More Than Sound).

37. David, S. (2016), *Emotional agility: Get unstuck, embrace change, and thrive in work and life* (New York: Avery), 1.

7. INVESTING IN A POSITIVE LEARNING ENVIRONMENT

1. Hammond, Z. (2015), *Culturally responsive teaching and the brain* (Thousand Oaks, CA: Sage); Staats, C. (2015), Understanding implicit bias: What educators should know, *American Educator*, retrieved fromhttp://www.aft.org/ae/winter2015-2016/staats; Tuckman, B. W., & Jensen, M. A. C. (1977), Stages of small group development revisited, *Group and Organizational Studies*, *2*(4), 419–427.

2. Aspen Institute (2018), *From a nation at risk to a nation at hope: Recommendations from the National Commission on Social, Emotional, & Academic Development* (Washington, DC: Aspen Institute), 17, retrieved fromhttp://nationathope.org/wp-content/uploads/2018_aspen_final-report_full_webversion.pdf

3. Collaborative for Academic, Social, and Emotional Learning (2019), Core SEL competencies, retrieved fromhttps://casel.org/core-competencies/

4. Schonert-Reichl, K. A. (2017), Social and emotional learning and teachers, *Future of Children*, *27*(1), 137–155; Schonert-Reichl, K. A., Kitil, M. J., & Hanson-Peterson, J. (2017), *To reach the students, teach the teachers: A national scan of teacher preparation and social and emotional learning: A report prepared for the Collaborative for Academic, Social, and Emotional Learning (CASEL)* (Vancouver, BC: University of British Columbia).

5. Jones, S. M., Bouffard, S. M., & Weissbourd, R. (2013), Educators' social and emotional skills vital to learning, *Phi Delta Kappan*, *94*(8), 63.

6. Collaborative for Academic, Social, and Emotional Learning, (2019), District resource center: SEL as a lever for equity, retrieved fromhttps://drc.casel.org/sel-as-a-lever-for-equity/

7. Immordino-Yang, M. H., Darling-Hammond, L., & Krone, C. (2018), *The brain basis for integrated social, emotional, and academic development: How emotions and social rela-*

tionships drive learning (Washington, DC: Aspen Institute), retrieved fromhttps://www.aspeninstitute.org/publications/the-brain-basis-for-integrated-social-emotional-and-academic-development/

8. Hammond, Z. (2015), *Culturally responsive teaching and the brain* (Thousand Oaks, CA: Sage); Hollins, E. R. (2008), *Culture in school learning: Revealing the deep meaning* (New York: Routledge); Staats, C. (2015), Understanding implicit bias: What educators should know, *American Educator*, retrieved fromhttp://www.aft.org/ae/winter2015-2016/staats

9. Berman, S., Chaffee, S., & Sarmiento, J. (2018), *The practice base for how we learn: Supporting students' social, emotional, and academic development* (Washington, DC: Aspen Institute), 8, retrieved fromhttps://assets.aspeninstitute.org/content/uploads/2018/03/CDE-Commission-report.pdf

10. Gaitan, C. D. (2006), *Building culturally responsive classrooms* (Thousand Oaks, CA: Sage).

11. Schonert-Reichl, Social and emotional learning, 139.

12. Tyng, C. M., Amin, H. U., Saad, M. N. M., & Malik, A. S. (2017), The influences of emotion on learning and memory, *Frontiers in Psychology*, 8, 1454.

13. Goleman, D., & Senge, P. (2014), *The triple focus: A new approach to education* (Florence, MA: More Than Sound), 16.

14. Kuhl, P. (2018, August 6), Masters of social learning, Aspen Institute [video file], retrieved fromhttps://www.aspeninstitute.org/videos/learning-and-the-social-brain/

15. Goleman, D. (2013), *Focus: The hidden driver of excellence* (New York: HarperCollins).

16. Medina, J. (2008), *Brain rules* (Seattle: Pear Press).

17. Goleman, *Focus*; Medina, *Brain rules*.

18. Nichols, J. D. (2011), *Teachers as servant leaders* (New York: Rowman & Littlefield).

19. Hammond, *Culturally responsive teaching*; Staats, C., & Contractor, D. (2014), *Race and discipline in Ohio schools: What the data say* (Columbus: Kirwan Institute for the Study of Race and Ethnicity at Ohio State University).

20. Nichols, *Teachers as servant leaders*.

21. Berger, R., Berman, S., Garcia, J., & Deasy, J. (2019), *A practice agenda in support of how learning happens* (Washington, DC: Aspen Institute), retrieved fromhttp://nationathope.org/research-practice-and-policy-agendas/practice/; Berman, Chaffee, & Sarmiento, *Practice base*.

22. Tuckman & Jensen, Small group development.

23. Fredrickson, B. L. (2013), Positive emotions broaden and build, *Advances in Experimental Social Psychology*, 47, 1–53; Kashdan, T., & Biswas-Diener, R. (2014), *The upside of your dark side* (New York: Penguin).

24. Fredrickson, B. L., & Branigan, C. (2005), Positive emotions broaden the scope of attention and thought-action repertoires, *Cognition and Emotion*, 19, 313–332; Lench, H. C., Flores, S. A., & Bench, S. W. (2011), Discrete emotions predict changes in cognition, judgment, experience, behavior, and physiology: A meta-analysis of experimental emotion elicitations, *Psychology Bulletin*, 137, 834–855.

25. Fredrickson, B. (2019), PEP lab, University of North Carolina at Chapel Hill, retrieved fromhttp://peplab.web.unc.edu/research/

26. Fredrickson, B. L. (1998), What good are positive emotions? *Review of General Psychology* [Special issue]. *New Directions in Research on Emotion*, 2(3), 300–319; Fredrickson, B. L. (2001), The role of positive emotions in positive psychology: The broaden-and-build theory of positive emotions, *American Psychologist*, 56, 218–226.

27. Fredrickson, PEP lab.

28. Fredrickson, Positive emotions broaden.
29. Fredrickson, PEP lab.

8. CONNECTING WITH PARENTS AND CAREGIVERS

1. Christenson, S. L., & Reschly, A. L. (2010), *Handbook of school–family partnerships* (New York: Routledge); Epstein, J. L. (2011), *School, family, and community partnerships: Preparing educators and improving schools* (Boulder, CO: Westview Press).

2. Collaborative for Academic, Social, and Emotional Learning (2019), Focus area 3: Family partnership, *Guide to schoolwide SEL*, retrieved fromhttps://schoolguide.casel.org/focus-area-3/family-partnerships/

3. Collaborative for Academic, Social, and Emotional Learning (2019), Core SEL competencies, retrieved fromhttps://casel.org/core-competenciess

9. RELATIONSHIPS WITH COLLEAGUES

1. Bryk, A. S., Bender Sebring, P., Allensworth, E., Luppescu, S., & Easton, J. Q. (2010), *Organizing schools for improvement: Lessons from Chicago* (Chicago: University of Chicago Press); Cranston, J. (2011), Relational trust: The glue that binds a professional learning community, *Alberta Journal of Educational Research*, 57(1), 59–72; Van Maele, D., & Van Houtte, M. (2015), Trust in school: A pathway to inhibit teacher burnout? *Journal of Educational Administration*, 53(1), 93–115.

2. Bryk, A. S., & Schneider, B. (2002), *Trust in schools: A core research for improvement* (New York: Russell Sage Foundation), 137.

3. Seppala, E. (2019, November 7), Four ways to calm your mind in stressful times, *Greater Good Magazine*, 7, retrieved fromhttps://greatergood.berkeley.edu/article/item/four_ways_to_calm_your_mind_in_stressful_times

4. Seppala, Four ways, 7.

5. Seppala, Four ways.

6. Jean Baker Miller Training Institute (2019), The development of Relational-Cultural Theory, retrieved fromhttps://www.wcwonline.org/JBMTI-Site/the-development-of-relational-cultural-theory

7. Jean Baker Miller Training Institute (2019), retrieved fromhttps://www.wcwonline.org/JBMTI-Site/introduction-to-jbmti

8. Collaborative for Academic, Social, and Emotional Learning (2019), Core SEL competencies, retrieved fromhttps://casel.org/core-competencies/

9. Edutopia (2018, February 5), Tap-in/tap-out: Giving teachers time to recharge [video file], retrieved fromhttps://www.youtube.com/watch?time_continue=84&v=qPtsP7pBobI

10. Richardson, P. W., Karabenick, S. A., & Watt, H. M. G. (Eds.) (2014), *Teacher motivation: Theory and practice* (New York: Taylor & Francis).

11. Evans, R. (1996), *The human side of school change: Reform, resistance, and the real-life problems of innovation* (San Francisco: Jossey-Bass); McGonigal, K. (2012), *The neuroscience of change* (Louisville, CO: Sounds True).

12. Hoerr, T. R. (2016), *The formative five: Fostering grit, empathy, and other success skills every student needs* (Alexandria, VA: ASCD); Martin, J. R. (2011), *Education reconfigured: Culture, encounter, and change* (New York: Routledge); Schmoker, M. (2016), *Leading with focus* (Alexandria, VA: ASCD).

13. Santoro, D. A. (2018), Is it burnout? Or demoralization? *Educational Leadership, 75*(6), 10.

14. Lopez, S. J. (2013), *Making hope happen* (New York: Simon & Shuster); Lopez, S. J., & Snyder, C. R. (2009), *The Oxford handbook of positive psychology* (New York: Oxford University Press).

15. Cited in Lopez, *Making hope happen*.

16. Rego, A., Machado, F., Leal, S., & Cunha, M. P. E. (2009), Are hopeful employees more creative? An empirical study, *Creativity Research Journal, 21*(2), 223–231.

17. Lopez, *Making hope happen*.

18. Rego, et al., Hopeful employees.

19. Becker, E. S., Goetz, T., Morger, V., & Ranellucci, J. (2014), The importance of teachers' emotions and instructional behavior for their students' emotions: An experience sampling analysis, *Teaching and Teacher Education, 43*, 15–26; Lopez, *Making hope happen*.

20. University of Minnesota (2013, May 7), An interview with Dr. Shane Lopez [video file], retrieved from https://www.youtube.com/watch?v=Bka3sI5_WZ4

21. Stavros, J., & Torres, C. (2018), *Conversations worth having* (Oakland, CA: Berrett-Koehler).

22. Collaborative for Academic, Social, and Emotional Learning (2019), Social and emotional learning 3 signature practices playbook, retrieved from https://drc.casel.org/blog/resource/sel-3-signature-practices-playbook-2/micro-sel-3-signature-practices-for-everyone-every-day/

23. Cooperrider, D. L. (2018), introduction, in J. Stavros & C. Torres, *Conversations worth having* (1–11) (Oakland, CA: Berrett-Koehler), 1.

24. Chabris, C. F., & Simons, D. J. (2010), *The invisible gorilla: And other ways our intuitions deceive us* (New York: Random House).

25. David, S. (2016), *Emotional agility: Get unstuck, embrace change, and thrive in work and life* (New York: Avery), 1.

26. Lambert, N. M., Gwinn, A. M., Baumeister, R. F., Strachman, A., Washburn, I. J., Gable, S. L., & Fincham, F. D. (2013), A boost of positive affect: The perks of sharing positive experiences, *Journal of Social and Personal Relationships, 30*(1), 24–43, cited in Hood, K. (2019), The benefits of active constructive responding, Institute of Positive Education, retrieved from https://www.ggs.vic.edu.au/blog-posts/the-benefits-of-active-constructive-responding

27. Gable, S. L., Reis, H. T., Impett, E. A., & Asher, E. R. (2004), What do you do when things go right? The intrapersonal and interpersonal benefits of sharing positive events, *Journal of Personality and Social Psychology, 87*(2), 228.

28. Scioli, A., & Biller, H. B. (2009), *Hope in the age of anxiety* (New York: Oxford University Press).

29. Bryk, A. S., & Schneider, B. (2003), Trust in schools: A core resource for school reform, *Educational Leadership, 60*(6), 40–45.

30. Bryk, A. S., & Schneider, B. (1996), *Social trust: A moral resource for school improvement* (Chicago: Consortium on Chicago School Research).

31. Van Maele & Van Houtte, Trust in school.

32. Cooperrider, introduction, 10.

10. THE ADMINISTRATION OF SCHOOLS

1. Berger, R., Berman, S., Garcia, J., & Deasy, J. (2019), *A practice agenda in support of how learning happens* (Washington, DC: Aspen Institute), 43, retrieved fromhttp://nationathope.org/research-practice-and-policy-agendas/practice/
2. Gable, S. L., & Bromberg, C. (2018), Healthy social bonds: A necessary condition for well-being, in E. Diener, S. Oishi, & L. Tay (Eds.), *Handbook of well-being* (Salt Lake City: DEF), 1.
3. Bryk, A. S., & Schneider, B. (2002), *Trust in schools: A core resource for improvement* (New York: Russell Sage Foundation), 139.
4. Bryk & Schneider, *Trust in schools*, 139.
5. Bryk & Schneider, *Trust in schools*, 139.
6. Bryk, A. S., & Schneider, B. (2003), Trust in schools: A core resource for school reform, *Educational Leadership*, 60(6), 42.
7. Bryk & Schneider, *Trust in schools*, 111.
8. Cranston, J. (2011), Relational trust: The glue that binds a professional learning community, *Alberta Journal of Educational Research*, 57(1), 59–72.
9. Cranston, Relational trust, 70.
10. Berger et al., *Practice agenda*, 18.
11. Becker, E. S., Goetz, T., Morger, V., & Ranellucci, J. (2014), The importance of teachers' emotions and instructional behavior for their students' emotions: An experience sampling analysis, *Teaching and Teacher Education*, 43, 15–26.
12. Mitchum, R. (2009, October 13), Laughing with your brain, *Science Life*, retrieved fromhttps://sciencelife.uchospitals.edu/2009/10/13/laughing-with-your-brain/
13. Becker et al., Importance of teachers' emotions.
14. Mitchum, Laughing with your brain.
15. Hanson, R. (2013), *Hardwiring happiness: The new brain science of contentment, calm, and confidence* (New York: Random House); Baumeister, R. F., Bratslavsky, E. Finkenauer, C., & Vohs, K. D. (2001), Bad is stronger than good, *Review of General Psychology*, 5(4), 323–370; Rozin, P., & Royzman, E. B. (2001), Negativity bias, negativity dominance, and contagion. *Personality and Social Psychology Review*, 5(4), 296–320.
16. Baumeister et al., Bad is stronger; Hanson, *Hardwiring happiness*.
17. Quoted in Thiers, N. (2016), Educators deserve better: A conversation with Richard DuFour, *Educational Leadership*, 73(8), 12.
18. Fiarman, S. E. (2015), *Becoming a school principal: Learning to lead, leading to learn*, Cambridge, MA: Harvard Education Press; Thiers, Educators deserve better.
19. Fiarman, S. (2017, July 19), Two things principals can do to support deeper learning, *Education Week*, retrieved fromhttp://blogs.edweek.org/edweek/learning_deeply/2017/07/two_things_principals_can_do_to_support_deeper_learning.html
20. Santoro, D. A. (2018), *Demoralized: Why teachers leave the profession they love and how they can stay* (Cambridge, MA: Harvard Education Press).
21. Santoro, D. A. (2018), Is it burnout? Or demoralization? *Educational Leadership*, 75(6), 10–15.
22. Cited in D'Orio, W. (2018, September 27), What's the difference between burnout and demoralization, and what can teachers do about it? *Education Weeks*, retrieved fromhttp://blogs.edweek.org/edweek/education_futures/2018/09/what_the_difference_between_burnout_and_demoralization_and_what_can_teachers_do_about_it.html
23. Cited in D'Orio, What's the difference?

24. Superville, D. R. (2019, December 19), Principal turnover is a problem: New data could help districts combat it, *Education Week*, retrieved fromhttps://www.edweek.org/ew/articles/2019/12/19/principal-turnover-is-a-problem-new-data.html

25. Bandura, A. (1993), Perceived self-efficacy in cognitive development and functioning, *Educational Psychologist*, *28*(2), 117–148; Donohoo, J., Hattie, J., & Eells, R. (2018), The power of collective efficacy, *Educational Leadership*, *75*(6), 40–44, 1.

26. Hattie, J. (2016, July), Mindframes and maximizers, third annual Visible Learning Conference, Washington, DC.

27. Donohoo, Hattie, & Eells, Power of collective efficacy, 40–44.

PERSONAL PRACTICES AND SKILLS

1. Horowitz, A. (2013), *On looking: A walker's guide to the art of observation* (New York: Scribner), 4.

11. CURIOSITY

1. Engel, S. (2015), *The hungry mind: The origins of curiosity in childhood* (Cambridge, MA: Harvard University Press), 10.

2. Kashdan, T. (2009), *Curious* (New York: HarperCollins); Opdal, P. M. (2001), Curiosity, wonder, and education seen as perspective development, *Studies in Philosophy and Education*, *20*(4), 331–344.

3. Hulme, E., Green, D. T., & Ladd, K. S. (2013), Fostering student engagement by cultivating curiosity, *New Directions for Student Services*, *2013*(143), 63.

4. Engel, *Hungry mind*, 16.

5. Berlyne, D. E. (1954), A theory of human curiosity, *British Journal of Psychology*, *45*(3), 180–191; Reio, T. G. (2008), Modeling curiosity, *New Horizons in Adult Education & Human Resource Development*, *22*(3/4), 3–5.

6. How curiosity enhances learning (2014, October 9), *Nature*, *514*(7521), 143.

7. Hulme, Green, & Ladd, Fostering student engagement.

8. Roman, B. (2011), Curiosity: A best practice in education, *Medical Education*, *45*(7), 654–656.

9. Engel, *Hungry mind*; Senge, P., Cambron-McCabe, N., Lucas, T., Smith, B., Dutton, J., & Kleiner, A. (2012), *Schools that learn* (New York: Random House).

10. Goodwin, B. (2014), Research says/curiosity is fleeting, but teachable, *Educational Leadership*, *72*(1), 73–74.

11. Hulme, Green, & Ladd, Fostering student engagement, 63.

12. Engel, *Hungry mind*; Hulme, Green, & Ladd, Fostering student engagement.

13. Brookfield, S. D. (2009), *The skillful teacher: On technique, trust, and responsiveness in the classroom* (San Francisco: Wiley); Langer, E. J. (2014), *Mindfulness* (Reading, MA: Addison-Wesley).

14. Tangney, J. P. (2000), Humility: Theoretical perspectives, empirical findings and directions for future research, *Journal of Social and Clinical Psychology*, *19*, 73–74.

15. Morgan, N. (2001, September 10), Do you have change fatigue? *Working Knowledge*, retrieved from https://hbswk.hbs.edu/item/do-you-have-change-fatigue

16. Bernerth, J. B., Walker, H. J., & Harris, S. G. (2011), Change fatigue: Development and initial validation of a new measure, *Work and Stress*, *25*(4), 321–337; Evans, R. (1996), *The human side of school change: Reform, resistance, and the real-life problems of innovation* (San Francisco: Jossey-Bass).

17. Phillips, D. K., & Carr, K. (2014), *Becoming a teacher through action research: Process, context, and self-study* (New York: Taylor & Francis); Saphier, J., Haley-Speca, M. A., & Gower, R. (2008), *The skillful teacher* (Acton, MA: Research for Better Teaching).

18. Hulme, Green, & Ladd, Fostering student engagement.

19. Larrivee, B. (2012), *Cultivating teacher renewal* (Plymouth, UK: Rowman & Littlefield).

20. Singer, J. (2010), *The teacher's ultimate stress mastery guide* (New York: Corwin).

21. Matta, C. (2012), *The stress response* (Oakland, CA: New Harbinger); Singer, *Teacher's ultimate stress mastery*.

22. McGonigal, K. (2015), *The upside of stress* (New York: Penguin); Singer, *Teacher's ultimate stress mastery*.

23. Achor, S. (2013), *Before happiness: The five hidden keys to achievement* (New York: Random House).

24. Reio, T. G. (2013), The cycle of curiosity, *New Horizons in Adult Education & Human Resource Development*, *25*(3), 1.

25. Kashdan, *Curious*.

26. Kashdan, T., & Steger, M. (2007), Curiosity and pathways to well-being and meaning in life: Traits, states, and everyday behaviors, *Motivation and Emotion*, *31*(3), 159–173; Reio, T. G., & Wiswell, A. (2000), Field investigation of the relationship among adult curiosity, workplace learning, and job performance, *Human Resource Development Quarterly*, *11*(1), 5–30; Swan, G. E., & Carmelli, D. (1996), Curiosity and mortality in aging adults: A 5-year follow-up of the western collaborative group study, *Psychology and Aging*, *11*(3), 449–453.

27. Hulme, Green, & Ladd, Fostering student engagement.

28. Kashdan, *Curious*; Opdal, Curiosity, wonder, and education.

12. REFLECTION

1. Brookfield, S. D. (2009), *The skillful teacher: On technique, trust, and responsiveness in the classroom* (San Francisco: Wiley); Kytle, J. (2004), *To want to learn* (New York: Palgrave Macmillan).

2. Cited in Cuban, L. (2011, June 16), Jazz, basketball, and teacher decision-making, *Larry Cuban on School Reform and Classroom Practice*, retrieved from https://larrycuban.wordpress.com/2011/06/16/jazz-basketball-and-teacher-decision-making/

3. Goleman, D. (2013), *Focus: The hidden driver of excellence* (New York: HarperCollins); Gün, B. (2014), Making sense of experienced teachers' interactive decisions: Implications for expertise in teaching, *International Journal of Instruction*, *7*(1), 75–90; Hyland, T. (2011), *Mindfulness and learning* (London: Springer).

4. Eberhardt, J. L. (2019), *Biased: Uncovering the hidden prejudice that shapes what we see, think, and do* (New York: Viking), 152.

5. Goleman, *Focus*.

6. McGonigal, K. (2015), *The upside of stress* (New York: Penguin).

7. Berman, S., Chaffee, S., & Sarmiento, J. (2018), *The practice base for how we learn: Supporting students' social, emotional, and academic development* (Washington, DC: Aspen Institute), retrieved fromhttps://assets.aspeninstitute.org/content/uploads/2018/03/CDE-Commission-report.pdf; Bridges, W. (1980), *Transitions* (New York: Addison-Wesley); Brookfield, S. (2017), *Becoming a critically reflective teacher*, 2nd ed. (San Francisco: Jossey-Bass); Brookfield, *Skillful teacher*; Collaborative for Academic, Social, and Emotional Learning (2019), Core SEL competencies, retrieved fromhttps://casel.org/core-competencies/; Engel, S. (2015), *The hungry mind: The origins of curiosity in childhood* (Cambridge, MA: Harvard University Press); Evans, R. (1996), *The human side of school change: Reform, resistance, and the real-life problems of innovation* (San Francisco: Jossey-Bass); Fredrickson, B. L. (2013), Positive emotions broaden and build, *Advances in Experimental Social Psychology*, 47, 1–53; Hammond, Z. (2015), *Culturally responsive teaching and the brain* (Thousand Oaks, CA: Sage); Kashdan, T. (2009), *Curious* (New York: HarperCollins); Kegan, R. (1982), *The evolving self* (Cambridge, MA: Harvard University Press); Mertler, C. A. (2014), *Action research* (Thousand Oaks, CA: Sage); Schwartz, H. L. (2019), *Connected teaching: Relationship, power, and mattering in higher education* (Sterling, VA: Stylus).

8. Goleman, D., & Senge, P. (2014), *The triple focus: A new approach to education* (Florence, MA: More Than Sound), 7.

9. Senge, P., Scharmer, C. O., Jaworski, J., & Flowers, B. S. (2004), *Presence: An exploration of profound change in people, organizations, and society* (New York: Random House).

10. Senge et al., *Presence*.

11. Goleman & Senge, *Triple focus*, 35.

12. Senge et al., *Presence*.

13. Pennebaker, J. W. (1997), *Opening up: The healing power of expressing emotions* (Boston: Guilford).

14. Expressive writing (2020), Greater Good in Action, retrieved fromhttps://ggia.berkeley.edu/practice/expressive_writing

15. Larrivee, B. (2012), *Cultivating teacher renewal* (Plymouth, UK: Rowman & Littlefield).

16. Staats, C. (2015), Understanding implicit bias: What educators should know, *American Educator*, retrieved fromhttp://www.aft.org/ae/winter2015-2016/staats; Staats, C., & Contractor, D. (2014), *Race and discipline in Ohio schools: What the data say* (Columbus: Kirwan Institute for the Study of Race and Ethnicity at Ohio State University).

17. Eberhardt, *Biased*, 6–7.

18. Staats, Understanding implicit bias; Staats & Contractor, *Race and discipline*.

19. Eberhardt, *Biased*, 302.

20. Benson, T. A., & Fiarman, S. E. (2019), *Unconscious bias in schools: A developmental approach to exploring race and racism* (Cambridge, MA: Harvard Education Press), 51.

21. Benson & Fiarman, *Unconscious bias*, 87.

22. Freemark, S. (2014, October 16), Studying with quizzes helps make sure the material sticks, Mindshift, retrieved fromhttps://www.kqed.org/mindshift/37752/studying-with-quizzes-helps-make-sure-the-material-sticks

23. Freemark, Studying with quizzes.

24. Hanson, R. (2013), *Hardwiring happiness: The new brain science of contentment, calm, and confidence* (New York: Random House).

25. Kashdan, T., & Biswas-Diener, R. (2014), *The upside of your dark side* (New York: Penguin).

26. Becker, E. S., Goetz, T., Morger, V., & Ranellucci, J. (2014), The importance of teachers' emotions and instructional behavior for their students' emotions: An experience sampling analysis, *Teaching and Teacher Education, 43*, 17.

27. Fredrickson, B. L. (2001), The role of positive emotions in positive psychology: The broaden-and-build theory of positive emotions, *American Psychologist, 56*, 218–226.

28. Devine, P., & Plant, A. (Eds.) (2013), *Advances in experimental social psychology* (Kidlington, UK: Academic Press), 45.

29. Lopez, S. J. (2013), *Making hope happen* (New York: Simon & Shuster).

13. PREPARATION AND SELF-CARE

1. Pasteur, L. (1854), Dans les champs de l'observation le hasard ne favorise que les esprits prepares, lecture, University of Lille, France.

2. Castro, A., Quinn, D. J., Fuller, E., & Barnes, M. (2018, January), *Policy brief 2018-1: Addressing the importance and scale of the U.S. teacher shortage*, UCEA Policy Briefs Series (Charlottesville, VA: University Council for Educational Administration).

3. Harris, B. (2015), *Retaining new teachers: How do I support and develop novice teachers?* (Alexandria, VA: ASCD/Arias).

4. Greenberg, M. T., Brown, J. L., & Abenavoli, R. M. (2016, September 1), Teacher stress and health: Effects on teachers, students, and schools, Robert Wood Johnson Foundation, 2, retrieved from http://prevention.psu.edu/uploads/files/rwjf430428.pdf

5. Smalley, S. L., & Winston, D. (2010), *Fully present: The science, art, and practice of mindfulness* (Philadelphia: Perseus).

6. Hyland, T. (2011), *Mindfulness and learning* (London: Springer), 63.

7. Flook, L., Goldberg, S. B., Pinger, L., Bonus, K., & Davidson, R. J. (2013), Mindfulness for teachers: A pilot study to assess effects on stress, burnout, and teaching efficacy, *International Mind, Brain, and Education, 7*(3), 182–195; Kabat-Zinn, J. (2005), *Coming to our senses: Healing ourselves and the world through mindfulness* (New York: Hyperion); Smalley & Winston, *Fully present*.

8. Goleman, D., & Senge, P. (2014), *The triple focus: A new approach to education* (Florence, MA: More Than Sound), 41.

9. Neff, K. (2011), *Self-compassion* (New York: HarperCollins).

10. Richardson, P. W., Karabenick, S. A., & Watt, H. M. G. (2014), *Teacher motivation: Theory and practice* (New York: Taylor & Francis); Saphier, J., Haley-Speca, M. A., & Gower, R. (2008), *The skillful teacher* (Acton, MA: Research for Better Teaching).

11. Baumeister, R. F., Bratslavsky, E., Finkenauer, C., & Vohs, K. D. (2001), Bad is stronger than good, *Review of General Psychology, 5*(4), 323–370.

12. Rozin, P., & Royzman, E. B. (2001), Negativity bias, negativity dominance, and contagion, *Personality and Social Psychology Review, 5*(4), 296–320.

13. Howells, K. (2012), *Gratitude in education: A radical view* (Boston: Sense); Palmer, P. (2007), *Courage to teach* (San Francisco: Jossey-Bass).

14. Nieto, S. (2003), *What keeps teachers going?* (New York: Teachers College Press), 24.

15. Howells, *Gratitude in education*.

16. Howells, *Gratitude in education*; Howells, K. (2014), An exploration of the role of gratitude in enhancing teacher–student relationships, *Teaching and Teacher Education, 42*, 58–67; Howells, K. (2015), Researching the place of gratitude in the personal domain of the

educator: Tales from the field. In K. Trimmer, A. L. Black, & S. Riddle (Eds.), *Mainstreams, margins, and the spaces in-between: New possibilities for education research* (36–49) (New York: Routledge); Lyubomirsky, S., & Kurtz, J. (2013), *Positively happy: Routes to sustainable happiness*, Positive Psychology Workbook Series (CreateSpace); Watkins, P. C. (2014), *Gratitude and the good life: Toward a psychology of appreciation* (New York: Springer).

17. Howells, K. (2012), *Gratitude in education*, 4.

14. WHAT MAKES GREAT TEACHERS GREAT?

1. Goleman, D. (1985), *Vital lies, simple truths: The psychology of self-deception* (New York: Simon & Schuster), 24.

2. Perspicacity (n.d.), *American Heritage Dictionary of the English Language*, Fifth Edition, retrieved from https://ahdictionary.com/word/search.html?q=perspicacity

3. Perspicacity (n.d.), *Vocabulary.com*, retrieved from https://www.vocabulary.com/dictionary/perspicacity

4. Scharmer, C. O. (2018), *The essentials of Theory U: Core principles and applications* (Oakland, CA: Berrett-Koehler).

5. Scharmer, *Essentials of Theory U*, 7–8.

6. Cuban, L. (2011, June 16), Jazz, basketball, and teacher decision-making, *Larry Cuban on School Reform and Classroom Practice*, retrieved from https://larrycuban.wordpress.com/2011/06/16/jazz-basketball-and-teacher-decision-making/

7. Brookfield, S. D. (2009), *The skillful teacher: On technique, trust, and responsiveness in the classroom* (San Francisco: Wiley); Eberhardt, J. L. (2019), *Biased: Uncovering the hidden prejudice that shapes what we see, think, and do* (New York: Viking).

8. Palmer, P. (2007), *Courage to teach* (San Francisco: Jossey-Bass).

9. Cullen, M., & Brito Pons, G. (2015), *The mindfulness-based emotional balance workbook* (Oakland, CA: New Harbinger); Howells, K. (2012), *Gratitude in education: A radical view* (Boston: Sense); Weng, H. Y., Fox, A. S., Shackman, A. J., Stodola, D. E., Caldwell, J. Z. K., Olson, M. C., Rogers, G. M, & Davidson, R. J. (2013), Compassion training alters altruism and neural responses to suffering, *Psychological science*, 24(7), 1171–1180.

10. Tangney J. P. (2000). Humility: Theoretical perspectives, empirical findings and directions for future research, *Journal of Social and Clinical Psychology*, 19, 73–74.

11. Goleman, D., & Senge, P. (2014), *The triple focus: A new approach to education* (Florence, MA: More Than Sound), 17–18.

12. David, S. (2016), *Emotional agility* (New York: Penguin Random House), 1.

13. Lopez, S. J. (2013), *Making hope happen* (New York: Simon & Shuster), 1.

14. Eberhardt, *Biased*, 143–144.

APPENDIX D. STANDPOINT EXPLORATION

1. Lee, C. (2014), In search of subjectivity: A reflection of a teacher educator in a cross-cultural context, *Educational Philosophy and Theory*, 46(13), 1427–1434; Smith, D. (1987), *The everyday world as problematic* (Boston: Northeastern University Press).

2. Chabris, C. F., & Simons, D. J. (2010), *The invisible gorilla: And other ways our intuitions deceive us* (New York: Random House); Eagleman, D. (2015), *The brain: The story of you* (New York: Penguin Random House); Simons, D. J. (2000), Attentional capture and inattentional blindness, *Trends in Cognitive Sciences, 4*(4), 147–155.

3. Smith, *Everyday world*.

4. Lee, In search of subjectivity; Smith, *Everyday world*.

5. Smith, *Everyday world*.

6. Lee, In search of subjectivity.

7. Richmond, G. (2019, October 28), The power of diversity, Sigma Xi, retrieved from https://www.sigmaxi.org/news/keyed-in/post/keyed-in/2019/10/28/the-power-of-diversity

APPENDIX E. EXPLORING HOPE

1. Lopez, S. J. (2013), *Making hope happen* (New York: Simon & Shuster).

2. Lopez, *Making hope happen*; Snyder, C. R. (2002), Hope theory: Rainbows in the mind, *Psychological Inquiry, 13*(4), 249–275.

3. Lopez, *Making hope happen*.

4. Lopez, *Making hope happen*.

5. McQuaid, M., & Lawn, E. (2014), *Your strengths blueprint: How to be engaged, energized, and happy at work* (Alberta Park, Australia: Version 2.0), 89.

6. Scioli, A., & Biller, H. B. (2009), *Hope in the age of anxiety* (New York: Oxford University Press), 18.

7. Lopez, *Making hope happen*.

8. Olson, K. (2014), *The invisible classroom: Relationships, neuroscience, and mindfulness in school* (New York: W. W. Norton).

9. Lopez, *Making hope happen*; Scioli & Biller, *Hope in the age*.

10. Evans, R. (1996), *The human side of school change: Reform, resistance, and the real-life problems of innovation* (San Francisco: Jossey-Bass).

11. Senge, P., Scharmer, C. O., Jaworski, J., & Flowers, B. S. (2004), *Presence: An exploration of profound change in people, organizations, and society* (New York: Random House).

12. Lopez, *Making hope happen*; Rego, A., Machado, F., Leal, S., & Cunha, M. P. E. (2009), Are hopeful employees more creative? An empirical study, *Creativity Research Journal, 21*(2), 223–231.

13. Lopez, *Making hope happen*; Rego et al., Hopeful employees.

14. Barsade, S. G. (2002), The ripple effect: Emotional contagion and its influence on group behavior, *Administrative Science Quarterly, 47*(4), 644–675; Hatfield, E., Cacioppo, J. T., Rapson, R. L. (1994), *Emotional contagion* (New York: Cambridge University Press); Lopez, *Making hope happen*.

15. Haskins, C. (2009), Teaching gratitude: Tools for inner peace and happiness, *Montessori Life, 21*(4), 26.

16. Lopez, *Making hope happen*.

17. Lopez, *Making hope happen*; Scioli & Biller, *Hope in the age*.

18. Scioli & Biller, *Hope in the age*.

19. Lopez, *Making hope happen*.

References

Achor, S. (2013). *Before happiness: The five hidden keys to achievement.* New York: Random House.

The Annie E. Casey Foundation Kids Count Data Center. (2020). Retrieved from http://datacenter.kidscount.org

Appiah, B. (2013, March 14). Selective attention and inattentional blindness: Test your awareness: Whodunnit? EdLab Columbia University. [Video file]. Retrieved from https://edlab.tc.columbia.edu/blog/9027-Selective-Attention-and-Inattentional-Blindness

Aspen Institute. (2018). *From a nation at risk to a nation at hope: Recommendations from the National Commission on Social, Emotional, and Academic Development.* Washington, DC: Aspen Institute. Retrieved from http://nationathope.org/wp-content/uploads/2018_aspen_final-report_full_webversion.pdf

Balonon-Rosen, P. (2016, January 7). Massachusetts education again ranks no. 1 nationally. Learning Lab. Retrieved from http://learninglab.legacy.wbur.org/2016/01/07/massachusetts-education-again-ranks-no-1-nationally/

Bandura, A. (1986). *Social foundations of thought and action: A social cognitive theory.* Englewood Cliffs, NJ: Prentice-Hall.

Bandura, A. (1993). Perceived self-efficacy in cognitive development and functioning. *Educational Psychologist, 28*(2), 117–148.

Barsade, S. G. (2002). The ripple effect: Emotional contagion and its influence on group behavior. *Administrative Science Quarterly, 47*(4), 644–675.

Baumeister, R. F., Bratslavsky, E., Finkenauer, C., & Vohs, K. D. (2001). Bad is stronger than good. *Review of General Psychology, 5*(4), 323–370.

Becker, E. S., Goetz, T., Morger, V., & Ranellucci, J. (2014). The importance of teachers' emotions and instructional behavior for their students' emotions: An experience sampling analysis. *Teaching and Teacher Education, 43,* 15–26.

Benson, T. A., & Fiarman, S. E. (2019). *Unconscious bias in schools: A developmental approach to exploring race and racism.* Cambridge, MA: Harvard Education Press.

Berardo, K., & Deardorff, D. (2012). *Building cultural competence: Innovative activities and models.* Sterling, VA: Stylus.

Berg, J. M., Dutton, J. E., & Wrzesniewski, A. (2013). Job crafting and meaningful work. In B. J. Dik., Z. S. Byrne, & M. F. Steger (Eds.). *Purpose and meaning in the workplace* (80–104). Washington, DC: American Psychological Association.

Berger, R., Berman, S., Garcia, J., & Deasy, J. (2019). *A practice agenda in support of how learning happens.* Washington, DC: Aspen Institute. Retrieved from http://nationathope.org/research-practice-and-policy-agendas/practice/

Berlyne, D. E. (1954). A theory of human curiosity. *British Journal of Psychology, 45*(3), 180–191.

Berman, S., Chaffee, S., & Sarmiento, J. (2018). *The practice base for how we learn: Supporting students' social, emotional, and academic development.* Washington, DC: Aspen Institute. Retrieved from https://assets.aspeninstitute.org/content/uploads/2018/03/CDE-Commission-report.pdf

Bernerth, J. B., Walker, H. J., & Harris, S. G. (2011). Change fatigue: Development and initial validation of a new measure. *Work and Stress, 25*(4), 321–337.

Bransford, J. D., Brown, A. L., & Cocking, R. R. (2000). *How people learn.* Washington, DC: National Academy Press.

Bridges, W. (1980). *Transitions.* New York: Addison-Wesley.

Brookfield, S. (2017). *Becoming a critically reflective teacher.* 2nd ed. San Francisco: Jossey-Bass.

Brookfield, S. D. (2009). *The skillful teacher: On technique, trust, and responsiveness in the classroom.* San Francisco: Wiley.

Bryk, A. S., Bender Sebring, P., Allensworth, E., Luppescu, S., & Easton, J. Q. (2010). *Organizing schools for improvement: Lessons from Chicago.* Chicago: University of Chicago Press.

Bryk, A. S., & Schneider, B. (1996). *Social trust: A moral resource for school improvement.* Chicago: Consortium on Chicago School Research.

Bryk, A. S., & Schneider, B. (2002). *Trust in schools: A core resource for improvement.* New York: Russell Sage Foundation.

Bryk, A. S., & Schneider, B. (2003). Trust in schools: A core resource for school reform. *Educational Leadership, 60*(6), 40–45.

Burnout. (n.d.). Lexico. Retrieved from https://en.oxforddictionaries.com/definition/burnout

Capp, M. J. (2017) The effectiveness of universal design for learning: A meta-analysis of literature between 2013 and 2016. *International Journal of Inclusive Education, 21*(8), 791–807.

Castro, A., Quinn, D. J., Fuller, E., & Barnes, M. (2018, January). *Policy brief 2018-1: Addressing the importance and scale of the U.S. teacher shortage.* UCEA Policy Briefs Series. Charlottesville, VA: University Council for Educational Administration.

Chabris, C. F., & Simons, D. J. (2010). *The invisible gorilla: And other ways our intuitions deceive us.* New York: Random House.

Chen, M., & Bargh, J. A. (1997). Nonconscious behavioral confirmation processes: The self-fulfilling consequences of automatic stereotype activation. *Journal of Experimental Social Psychology, 33,* 541–560.

Christenson, S. L., & Reschly, A. L. (2010). *Handbook of school-family partnerships.* New York: Routledge.

Collaborative for Academic, Social, and Emotional Learning. (2019). *Core SEL Competencies.* Retrieved from https://casel.org/core-competencies/

Collaborative for Academic, Social, and Emotional Learning. (2019). *District resource center: SEL as a lever for equity.* Retrieved from https://drc.casel.org/sel-as-a-lever-for-equity/

Collaborative for Academic, Social, and Emotional Learning. (2019). Focus area 3: Family partnership. *Guide to schoolwide SEL.* Retrieved from https://schoolguide.casel.org/focus-area-3/family-partnerships/

Collaborative for Academic, Social, and Emotional Learning. (2019). *SEL 3 signature practices playbook.* Retrieved from https://drc.casel.org/blog/resource/sel-3-signature-practices-playbook-2/micro-sel-3-signature-practices-for-everyone-every-day/

Cooperrider, D. L. (2018). Introduction. In J. Stavros & C. Torres. *Conversations worth having* (2–11). Oakland, CA: Berrett-Koehler.

Cranston, J. (2011). Relational trust: The glue that binds a professional learning community. *Alberta Journal of Educational Research, 57*(1), 59–72.

Creswell, J. W. (2008). *Educational research: Planning, conducting, and evaluating quantitative and qualitative research.* Upper Saddle River, NJ: Pearson.

Cuban, L. (2011, June 16). Jazz, basketball, and teacher decision-making. *Larry Cuban on School Reform and Classroom Practice.* Retrieved from https://larrycuban.wordpress.com/2011/06/16/jazz-basketball-and-teacher-decision-making/

Cullen, M., & Brito Pons, G. (2015). *The mindfulness-based emotional balance workbook.* Oakland, CA: New Harbinger.

David, S. (2016). *Emotional agility: Get unstuck, embrace change, and thrive in work and life.* New York: Avery.

Deal, T. E. & Kennedy, A. A. (1983, February). Culture and school performance. *Educational Leadership, 40*(5), 14–15.

Devine, P., & Plant, A. (Eds.). (2013). *Advances in experimental social psychology.* Kidlington, UK: Academic Press.

Dik, B. J., Byrne, Z. S., & Steger, M. F. (Eds.). (2013). *Purpose and meaning in the workplace.* Washington, DC: American Psychological Association.

Donohoo, J., Hattie, J., & Eells, R. (2018). The power of collective efficacy. *Educational Leadership, 75*(6), 40–44.

D'Orio, W. (2018, September 27). What's the difference between burnout and demoralization, and what can teachers do about it? *Education Weeks.* Retrieved from http://blogs.edweek.org/edweek/education_futures/2018/09/what_the_difference_between_burnout_and_demoralization_and_what_can_teachers_do_about_it.html

Dweck, C. (2000). *Self-theories.* Philadelphia: Taylor & Francis.

Dweck, C. S. (2006). *Mindset: The new psychology of success.* New York: Random House.

Eagleman, D. (2015). *The brain: The story of you.* New York: Penguin Random House.

Eberhardt, J. L. (2019). *Biased: Uncovering the hidden prejudice that shapes what we see, think, and do.* New York: Viking.

Edutopia. (2018, February 5). Tap-in/tap-out: Giving teachers time to recharge. [Video file]. Retrieved from https://www.youtube.com/watch?time_continue=84&v=qPtsP7pBobI

Edwards, C., Edwards, A., Torrens, A., & Beck, A. (2011). Confirmation and community—the relationships between teacher confirmation, classroom community, student motivation, and learning. *Online Journal of Communication and Media, 1*(4), 17–43. Retrieved from https://www.ojcmt.net/volume-1/issue-4

Engel, S. (2015). *The hungry mind: The origins of curiosity in childhood.* Cambridge, MA: Harvard University Press.

Epstein, J. L. (2011). *School, family, and community partnerships: Preparing educators and improving schools.* Boulder, CO: Westview Press.

Evans, R. (1996). *The human side of school change: reform, resistance, and the real-life problems of innovation.* San Francisco: Jossey-Bass.

Expressive writing. (2020). Greater Good in Action. Retrieved from https://ggia.berkeley.edu/practice/expressive_writing

Fiarman, S. E. (2015). *Becoming a school principal: Learning to lead, leading to learn.* Cambridge, MA: Harvard Education Press.

Fiarman, S. E. (2017, July 19). Two things principals can do to support deeper learning. *Education Week.* Retrieved from http://blogs.edweek.org/edweek/learning_deeply/2017/07/two_things_principals_can_do_to_support_deeper_learning.html

Fisher, B. (1991). *Joyful learning in kindergarten.* Portsmouth, NH: Heinemann.

Flook, L., Goldberg, S. B., Pinger, L., Bonus, K., & Davidson, R. J. (2013) Mindfulness for teachers: A pilot study to assess effects on stress, burnout, and teaching efficacy. *International Mind, Brain, and Education, 7*(3), 182–195.

Fredrickson, B. (2019). PEP lab. University of North Carolina at Chapel Hill. Retrieved from http://peplab.web.unc.edu/research/

Fredrickson, B. L. (1998). What good are positive emotions? *Review of General Psychology* [Special Issue]. *New Directions in Research on Emotion, 2*(3), 300–319.

Fredrickson, B. L. (2001). The role of positive emotions in positive psychology: The broaden-and-build theory of positive emotions. *American Psychologist, 56,* 218–226.

Fredrickson, B. L. (2013). Positive emotions broaden and build. *Advances in Experimental Social Psychology, 47,* 1–53.

Fredrickson, B. L., & Branigan, C. (2005). Positive emotions broaden the scope of attention and thought-action repertoires. *Cognition and Emotion, 19,* 313–332.

Freemark, S. (2014, October 16). Studying with quizzes helps make sure the material sticks. Mindshift. Retrieved from https://www.kqed.org/mindshift/37752/studying-with-quizzes-helps-make-sure-the-material-sticks

Frost, P., Casey, B., Griffin, K., Raymundo, L., Farrell, C., & Carrigan, R. (2015) The influence of confirmation bias on memory and source monitoring. *Journal of General Psychology, 142*(4), 238–252.

Gable, S. L., & Bromberg, C. (2018). Healthy social bonds: A necessary condition for well-being. In E. Diener, S. Oishi, & L. Tay (Eds.). *Handbook of well-being.* Salt Lake City: DEF.

Gable, S. L., Reis, H. T., Impett, E. A., & Asher, E. R. (2004). What do you do when things go right? The intrapersonal and interpersonal benefits of sharing positive events. *Journal of Personality and Social Psychology, 87*(2), 228.

Gaitan, C. D. (2006). *Building culturally responsive classrooms.* Thousand Oaks, CA: Sage.

Garner, P. W., Bender, S. L., & Fedor, M. (2018). Mindfulness-based SEL programming to increase preservice teachers' mindfulness and emotional competence. *Psychology in the Schools, 55*(4), 377–390.

Gay, G. (2010). *Culturally responsive teaching.* New York: Teachers College.

Goleman, D. (1985). *Vital lies, simple truths: The psychology of self-deception.* New York: Simon & Schuster.

Goleman, D. (2006). *Social intelligence: The new science of human relationships.* New York: Bantam Dell.

Goleman, D. (2013). *Focus: The hidden driver of excellence.* New York: HarperCollins.

Goleman, D., & Senge, P. (2014). *The triple focus: A new approach to education.* Florence, MA: More Than Sound.

Goodwin, B. (2014). Research says/curiosity is fleeting, but teachable. *Educational Leadership, 72*(1), 73–74.

Grant, A. (2018, November 12). Who we are: Collaborators. Ethical Systems. Retrieved from https://www.ethicalsystems.org/content/who-we-are

Greenberg, M. T., Brown, J. L., & Abenavoli, R. M. (2016, September 1). Teacher stress and health effects on teachers, students, and schools. Robert Wood Johnson Foundation. Retrieved from http://prevention.psu.edu/uploads/files/rwjf430428.pdf

Gregory, M., & Gregory, M. V. (2013). *Teaching excellence in higher education.* New York: Palgrave Macmillan.

Groccia, J. E. (2018, Summer). What is student engagement. *New Directions for Teaching and Learning, 154,* 11–20.

Guest, G., Bunce, A., & Johnson, L. (2006). How many interviews are enough? An experiment with data saturation and variability. *Field Methods, 18*(1), 59–82.

Gün, B. (2014). Making sense of experienced teachers' interactive decisions: Implications for expertise in teaching. *International Journal of Instruction, 7*(1), 75–90.

Gunderson, C., Graff, D., & Craddock, K. (Eds.). (2018). *Transforming community: Stories of connection through the lens of relational-cultural theory.* Duluth, MN: Whole Person.

Hammond, Z. (2015). *Culturally responsive teaching and the brain.* Thousand Oaks, CA: Sage.

Hanson, R. (2013). *Hardwiring happiness: The new brain science of contentment, calm, and confidence.* New York: Random House.

Harris, B. (2015). *Retaining new teachers: How do I support and develop novice teachers?* Alexandria, VA: ASCD/Arias.

Haskins, C. (2009). Teaching gratitude: Tools for inner peace and happiness. *Montessori Life, 21*(4), 26–32.

Hatfield, E., Cacioppo, J. T., & Rapson, R. L. (1994). *Emotional contagion.* New York: Cambridge University Press.

Hattie, J. (2016, July). Mindframes and maximizers. Third annual Visible Learning conference. Washington, DC.

Herman, K. C., Hickmon-Rosa, J., & Reinke, W. M. (2018). Empirically derived profiles of teacher stress, burnout, self-efficacy, and coping and associated student outcomes. *Journal of Positive Behavior Interventions, 20*(2), 90–100.

Hirshberg, M. J., Flook, L., Enright, R. D., & Davidson, R. J. (2020, April). Integrating mindfulness and connection practices into preservice teacher education improves classroom practices. *Learning and Instruction, 66,* 101298.

Hoerr, T. R. (2016). *The formative five: Fostering grit, empathy, and other success skills every student needs.* Alexandria, VA: ASCD.

Hood, K. (2019). The benefits of active constructive responding. Institute of Positive Education. Retrieved from https://www.ggs.vic.edu.au/blog-posts/the-benefits-of-active-constructive-responding

Hollins, E. R. (2008). *Culture in school learning: Revealing the deep meaning.* New York: Routledge.

Horowitz, A. (2013). *On looking: A walker's guide to the art of observation.* New York: Scribner.

How curiosity enhances learning. (2014, October 9) *Nature, 514*(7521), 143.

Howells, K. (2012). *Gratitude in education: A radical view.* Boston: Sense.

Howells, K. (2014). An exploration of the role of gratitude in enhancing teacher-student relationships. *Teaching and Teacher Education, 42,* 58–67.

Howells, K. (2015). Researching the place of gratitude in the personal domain of the educator: Tales from the field. In K. Trimmer, A. L. Black, & S. Riddle (Eds.). *Mainstreams, margins, and the spaces in-between: New possibilities for education research* (36–49). New York: Routledge.

Hulme, E., Green, D. T. & Ladd, K. S. (2013). Fostering student engagement by cultivating curiosity. *New Directions for Student Services, 2013*(143), 53–64.

Hyland, T. (2011). *Mindfulness and learning.* London: Springer.

Immordino-Yang, M. H., Darling-Hammond, L., & Krone, C. (2018). *The brain basis for integrated social, emotional, and academic development: How emotions and social relationships drive learning.* Washington, DC: Aspen Institute. Retrieved from https://www.aspeninstitute.org/publications/the-brain-basis-for-integrated-social-emotional-and-academic-development/

Jacobs, H. H. (2010). *Curriculum 21: Essential education for a changing world.* Alexandria, VA: ASCD.

Jean Baker Miller Training Institute. (2019). Retrieved from https://www.wcwonline.org/JBMTI-Site/introduction-to-jbmti

Jean Baker Miller Training Institute (2019). The development of Relational-Cultural Theory. Retrieved from https://www.wcwonline.org/JBMTI-Site/the-development-of-relational-cultural-theory

Jenko, M. (2014, March 13). EBP lecture for module 3: Qualitative designs, descriptive statistics. Retrieved from https://www.youtube.com/watch?v=ooNQmha-3Bw

Jennings, P. A., Frank, J. L., Snowberg, K. E., Coccia, M. A., & Greenberg, M. T. (2013). Improving classroom learning environments by cultivating awareness and resilience in education (CARE): Results of a randomized controlled trial. *School Psychology Quarterly*, *28*(4), 374–390.

Jones, S. M., Bouffard, S. M., & Weissbourd, R. (2013). Educators' social and emotional skills vital to learning. *Phi Delta Kappan*, *94*(8), 62–65.

Jordan, J. V. (2017, October). Relational-Cultural Theory: The power of connection to transform our lives. *Journal of Humanistic Counseling*, *56*(3), 228–240.

Jupp, J. C. (2013). *Becoming teachers of inner-city students: Life histories and teacher stories of committed white teachers.* Rotterdam, Netherlands: Sense.

Kabat-Zinn, J. (2005). *Coming to our senses: Healing ourselves and the world through mindfulness.* New York: Hyperion.

Kashdan, T. (2009). *Curious.* New York: HarperCollins.

Kashdan, T., & Biswas-Diener, R. (2014). *The upside of your dark side.* New York: Penguin.

Kashdan, T., & Steger, M. (2007). Curiosity and pathways to well-being and meaning in life: Traits, states, and everyday behaviors. *Motivation and Emotion*, *31*(3), 159–173.

Kegan, R. (1982). *The evolving self.* Cambridge, MA: Harvard University Press.

Kober, N. (2015). *Reaching students: What research says about effective instruction in undergraduate science and engineering.* Washington, DC: National Academies Press.

Kozak, A. (2009). *Wild chickens and petty tyrants: 108 metaphors for mindfulness.* Somerville, MA: Wisdom.

Kuhl, P. (2018, August 6). Masters of social learning. Aspen Institute. [Video file]. Retrieved from https://www.aspeninstitute.org/videos/learning-and-the-social-brain/

Kytle, J. (2004). *To want to learn.* New York: Palgrave Macmillan.

Lambert, N. M., Gwinn, A. M., Baumeister, R. F., Strachman, A., Washburn, I. J., Gable, S. L., & Fincham, F. D. (2013). A boost of positive affect: The perks of sharing positive experiences. *Journal of Social and Personal Relationships*, *30*(1), 24–43.

Langer, E. J. (2014). *Mindfulness.* Reading, MA: Addison-Wesley.

Larrivee, B. (2012). *Cultivating teacher renewal.* Plymouth, UK: Rowman & Littlefield.

Lee, C. (2014). In search of subjectivity: A reflection of a teacher educator in a cross-cultural context. *Educational Philosophy and Theory*, *46*(13), 1427–1434.

Lench, H. C., Flores, S. A., & Bench, S. W. (2011). Discrete emotions predict changes in cognition, judgment, experience, behavior, and physiology: A meta-analysis of experimental emotion elicitations. *Psychology Bulletin*, *137*, 834–855.

Levy, S. (1996). *Starting from scratch: One classroom builds its own curriculum*. Portsmouth, NH: Heinemann.
Lieberman, M. D. (2014). *Social: Why our brains are wired to connect*. New York: Crown.
Lopez, S. J. (2013). *Making hope happen*. New York: Simon & Shuster.
Lopez, S. J., & Snyder, C. R. (2009). *The Oxford handbook of positive psychology*. New York: Oxford University Press.
Lyubomirsky, S., & Kurtz, J. (2013). *Positively happy: Routes to sustainable happiness*. Positive Psychology Workbook Series. CreateSpace.
Mahoney, H. M. (2017, August 2). The other side of empathy. Medium. Retrieved from https://medium.com/stanford-d-school/the-other-side-of-empathy-6c1512aa2963
Martin, J. R. (2011). *Education reconfigured: Culture, encounter, and change*. New York: Routledge.
Mason, B. A., Gunersel, A. B., & Ney, E. A. (2014). Cultural and ethnic bias in teacher ratings of behavior: A criterion-focused review. *Psychology in the Schools, 51*(10), 1017–1030.
Massachusetts Department of Education. (2016). Enrollment by grade. Retrieved from http://profiles.doe.mass.edu/state_report/enrollmentbygrade.aspx
Massachusetts Department of Education. (2018). Educator evaluation. Retrieved from http://www.doe.mass.edu/edeval/resources/rubrics/
Massachusetts Department of Education. (2018). Educator evaluation data 2015–2016. Retrieved from http://profiles.doe.mass.edu/statereport/educatorevaluationperformance.aspx
Massachusetts earns a B-Plus on state report card, ranks first in nation. (2018, January 17). *Education Week*. Retrieved from https://www.edweek.org/ew/collections/quality-counts-2018-state-grades/highlight-reports/2018/01/17/massachusetts.html
Massachusetts Model System for Educator Evaluation (2015, December). *Part III: Guide to rubrics and model rubrics for superintendent, administrator, and teacher*. Malden: Massachusetts Department of Elementary and Secondary Education.
Matta, C. (2012). *The stress response*. Oakland, CA: New Harbinger.
McGonigal, K. (2012). *The neuroscience of change*. Louisville, CO: Sounds True.
McGonigal, K. (2015). *The upside of stress*. New York: Penguin.
McGrath, H., & Noble, T. (2010). Supporting positive pupil relationships: Research to practice. *Education & Child Psychology, 27*(1), 79–90.
McNerney, S. (2011). Confirmation bias and art. *Scientific American*. Retrieved from http://blogs.scientificamerican.com/guest-blog/confirmation-bias-and-art/
McQuaid, M., & Lawn, E. (2014). *Your strengths blueprint: How to be engaged, energized, and happy at work*. Alberta Park, Australia: Version 2.0.
Medina, J. (2008). *Brain rules*. Seattle: Pear Press.
Merriam, S. B. (2009). *Qualitative research: A guide to design and implementation*. San Francisco: Jossey-Bass.
Mertler, C. A. (2014). *Action research*. Thousand Oaks, CA: Sage.
Miller, J. B. (1976). *Toward a new psychology of women*. Boston: Beacon Press.
Miller, J. B. (1986). *What do we mean by relationships?* Work in Progress, no. 22. Wellesley, MA: Stone Center Working Paper Series.
Miller, J. B. (2008). How change happens: Controlling images, mutuality, and power. *Women & Therapy, 31*(2–4), 109–127.
Milner, R. H. (2011, January/February). Five easy ways to connect with students. *Harvard Education Letter, 27*(1).
Mitchum, R. (2009, October 13). Laughing with your brain. *Science Life*. Retrieved from https://sciencelife.uchospitals.edu/2009/10/13/laughing-with-your-brain/

Morgan, N. (2001, September 10). Do you have change fatigue? Working Knowledge. Retrieved from https://hbswk.hbs.edu/item/do-you-have-change-fatigue

Munoz, L. M. P. (2013, June 24). Feeling others' pain: Transforming empathy into compassion. Cognitive Neuroscience Society. Retrieved from https://www.cogneurosociety.org/empathy_pain/

Neault, R. A. (Ed.). (2011). *Thoughts on theories* [Special issue]. *Journal of Employment Counseling, 48*(4).

Neff, K. (2011). *Self-compassion*. New York: HarperCollins.

Nichols, J.D. (2011). *Teachers as servant leaders*. New York: Rowman & Littlefield.

Nickerson, R. S. (1998). Confirmation bias: A ubiquitous phenomenon in many guises. *Review of General Psychology, 2*(2), 175–220.

Niemiec, R. M. (2018). *Character strengths interventions: A field guide*. Boston: Hogrefe.

Niemiec, R. M., & McGrath, R. E. (2019). *The power of character strengths: Appreciate and ignite your positive personality*. Cincinnati, OH: VIA Institute on Character.

Nieto, S. (2003). *What keeps teachers going?* New York: Teachers College Press.

Olson, K. (2014). *The invisible classroom: Relationships, neuroscience, and mindfulness in school*. New York: W. W. Norton.

Opdal, P. M. (2001). Curiosity, wonder, and education seen as perspective development. *Studies in Philosophy and Education, 20*(4), 331–344.

Palmer, P. (2007). *Courage to teach*. San Francisco: Jossey-Bass.

Pasteur, L. (1854). Dans les champs de l'observation le hasard ne favorise que les esprits prepares. Lecture. University of Lille, France.

Pennebaker, J. W. (1997). *Opening up: The healing power of expressing emotions*. Boston: Guilford.

Phillips, D. K., & Carr, K. (2014). *Becoming a teacher through action research: Process, context, and self-study*. New York: Taylor & Francis.

Pielmeier, M., Huber, S., & Seidel, T. (2018). Is teacher judgment accuracy of students' characteristics beneficial for verbal teacher-student interactions in the classroom? *Teaching and Teacher Education, 76*(11), 255–266.

Pope, R. L., Reynolds, A. L., & Mueller, J. A. (2014). *Creating multicultural change on campus*. San Francisco: Jossey-Bass.

Rego, A., Machado, F., Leal, S., & Cunha, M. P. E. (2009). Are hopeful employees more creative? An empirical study. *Creativity Research Journal, 21*(2), 223–231.

Reio, T. G. (2008). Modeling curiosity. *New Horizons in Adult Education & Human Resource Development, 22*(3/4), 3–5.

Reio, T. G. (2013). The cycle of curiosity. *New Horizons in Adult Education & Human Resource Development, 25*(3), 1–2.

Reio, T. G., & Wiswell, A. (2000). Field investigation of the relationship among adult curiosity, workplace learning, and job performance. *Human Resource Development Quarterly, 11*(1), 5–30.

Richardson, P. W., Karabenick, S. A., & Watt, H. M. G. (Eds.). (2014). *Teacher motivation: Theory and practice*. New York: Taylor & Francis.

Richmond, G. (2019, October 28). The power of diversity. Sigma Xi. Retrieved from https://www.sigmaxi.org/news/keyed-in/post/keyed-in/2019/10/28/the-power-of-diversity

Roman, B. (2011). Curiosity: A best practice in education. *Medical Education, 45*(7), 654–656.

Rozin, P., & Royzman, E. B. (2001). Negativity bias, negativity dominance, and contagion. *Personality and Social Psychology Review, 5*(4), 296–320.

Salzberg, S. (2014). *Real happiness at work*. New York: Workman.

Santoro, D. (2011). Good teaching in difficult times: Demoralization in the pursuit of good work. *American Journal of Education, 118*(1), 1–23.

Santoro, D. A. (2018). *Demoralized: Why teachers leave the profession they love and how they can stay*. Cambridge, MA: Harvard Education Press.

Santoro, D. A. (2018). Is it burnout? Or demoralization? *Educational Leadership, 75*(6), 10–15.

Saphier, J., Haley-Speca, M. A., & Gower, R. (2008). *The skillful teacher*. Acton, MA: Research for Better Teaching.

Scharmer, C. O. (2018). *The essentials of Theory U: Core principles and applications*. Oakland, CA: Berrett-Koehler.

Schlechty, P. C. (2001). *Shaking up the schoolhouse: How to support and sustain educational innovation*. San Francisco: Jossey-Bass.

Schmidt, R. F. (1986). *Fundamentals of sensory physiology*. New York: Springer.

Schmoker, M. (2016). *Leading with focus*. Alexandria, VA: ASCD.

Schonert-Reichl, K. A. (2017). Social and emotional learning and teachers. *Future of Children, 27*(1), 137–155.

Schonert-Reichl, K. A., Kitil, M. J., & Hanson-Peterson, J. (2017). *To reach the students, teach the teachers: A national scan of teacher preparation and social and emotional learning*. A report prepared for the Collaborative for Academic, Social, and Emotional Learning (CASEL). Vancouver: University of British Columbia.

Schonert-Reichl, K. A., Oberle, E., Lawlor, M. S., Abbott, D., Thomson, K., Oberlander, T. F., & Diamond, A. (2015). Enhancing cognitive and social-emotional development through a simple-to-administer mindfulness-based school program for elementary school children: A randomized controlled trial. *Developmental Psychology, 51*(1), 52–66.

Schwartz, H. L. (2019). *Connected teaching: Relationship, power, and mattering in higher education*. Sterling, VA: Stylus.

Scioli, A., & Biller, H. B. (2009). *Hope in the age of anxiety*. New York: Oxford University Press.

Senge, P., Cambron-McCabe, N., Lucas, T., Smith, B., Dutton, J., & Kleiner, A. (2012). *Schools that learn: A fifth discipline fieldbook for educators, parents, and everyone who cares about education*. New York: Random House.

Senge, P., Scharmer, C. O., Jaworski, J., & Flowers, B. S. (2004). *Presence: An exploration of profound change in people, organizations, and society*. New York: Random House.

Seppala, E. (2019, November 7). Four ways to calm your mind in stressful times. *Greater Good Magazine*. Retrieved from https://greatergood.berkeley.edu/article/item/four_ways_to_calm_your_mind_in_stressful_times

Siblinga, E. M. S., Webb, L., Ghazarian, S. R., & Ellen, J. M. (2016). School-based mindfulness instruction: An RCT. *Pediatrics, 137*(1), 1–8.

Siegel, D. J. (2010). *Mindsight: The new science of personal transformation*. New York: Random House.

Simons, D. J. (2000). Attentional capture and inattentional blindness. *Trends in Cognitive Sciences, 4*(4), 147–155.

Simons, D. J., & Chabris, C. F. (1999) Gorillas in our midst: Sustained inattentional blindness for dynamic events. *Perception, 28*, 1059–1074.

Singer, J. (2010). *The teacher's ultimate stress mastery guide*. New York: Corwin.

Singer, T., & Bolz, M. (Eds.). (2014) *Compassion: Bridging practice and science*. Munich, Germany: Max Planck Society.

Sizer, T. R., & Faust Sizer, N. (1999). *The students are watching: Schools and the moral contract*. Boston: Beacon Press.

Smalley, S. L., & Winston, D. (2010). *Fully present: The science, art, and practice of mindfulness*. Philadelphia: Perseus.

Smith, D. (1987). *The everyday world as problematic*. Boston: Northeastern University Press.

Snyder, C. R. (2002). Hope theory: Rainbows in the mind. *Psychological Inquiry*, *13*(4), 249–275.

Split, J. L., Koomen, H. M. Y., & Thijs, J. T. (2011). Teacher wellbeing: The importance of teacher-student relationships. *Educational Psychology Review*, *23*(4), 457–477.

Staats, C. (2015) Understanding implicit bias: What educators should know. *American Educator.*. Retrieved from http://www.aft.org/ae/winter2015-2016/staats

Staats, C., & Contractor, D. (2014). *Race and discipline in Ohio schools: What the data say*. Columbus: Kirwan Institute for the Study of Race and Ethnicity at Ohio State University.

Stavros, J., & Torres, C. (2018). *Conversations worth having*. Oakland, CA: Berrett-Koehler.

Strouse, J. H. (2001). *Exploring socio-cultural themes in education*. Columbus, OH: Prentice-Hall.

Style, E. J. (2014). Curriculum as encounter: Selves and shelves. *English Journal*, *103*(5), 67–74.

Superville, D. R. (2019, December 19). Principal turnover is a problem: New data could help districts combat it. *Education Week*. Retrieved from https://www.edweek.org/ew/articles/2019/12/19/principal-turnover-is-a-problem-new-data.html

Surrey, J., & Kramer, G. (2013). Relational mindfulness. In C. K. Germer, R. D. Siegel, & P. R. Fulton (Eds.). *Mindfulness and psychotherapy* (94–111). New York: Guilford.

Swan, G. E., & Carmelli, D. (1996). Curiosity and mortality in aging adults: A 5-year follow-up of the western collaborative group study. *Psychology and Aging*, *11*(3), 449–453.

Tangney J. P. (2000). Humility: Theoretical perspectives, empirical findings and directions for future research. *Journal of Social and Clinical Psychology*, *19*, 70–82.

Taxer, J. L., Becker-Kurz, B., & Frenzel, A. C. (2019, February). Do quality teacher-student relationships protect teachers from emotional exhaustion? The mediating role of enjoyment and anger. *Social Psychology of Education*, *22*(1), 209–226.

Thiers, N. (2016). Educators deserve better: A conversation with Richard DuFour. *Educational Leadership*, *73*(8), 10–16.

Tuckman, B. W., & Jensen, M. A. C. (1977). Stages of small group development revisited. *Group and Organizational Studies*, *2*(4), 419–427.

Tyng, C. M., Amin, H. U., Saad, M. N. M., & Malik, A. S. (2017). The influences of emotion on learning and memory. *Frontiers in Psychology*, *8*, 1454.

University of Minnesota. (2013, May 7). An interview with Dr. Shane Lopez. [Video file]. Retrieved from https://www.youtube.com/watch?v=Bka3sI5_WZ4

Van Maele, D., & Van Houtte, M., (2015). Trust in school: A pathway to inhibit teacher burnout? *Journal of Educational Administration*, *53*(1), 93–115.

Walker, M. (2004). How relationships heal. In M. Walker & W. B. Rosen (Eds.). *How connections heal: Stories from Relational-Cultural Therapy* (3–21). New York: Guilford Press.

Walker, T. (2018, May 11). How many teachers are highly stressed? Maybe more people than your think. *NEA Today*. Retrieved from http://neatoday.org/2018/05/11/study-high-teacher-stress-levels/

Watkins, P. C. (2014). *Gratitude and the good life: Toward a psychology of appreciation*. New York: Springer.

Weng, H. Y., Fox, A. S., Shackman, A. J., Stodola, D. E., Caldwell, J. Z. K., Olson, M. C., Rogers, G. M., &Davidson, R. J. (2013). Compassion training alters altruism and neural responses to suffering. *Psychological Science*, *24*(7), 1171–1180.

Wrzesniewski, A. (2014, November 10). Job crafting: How individuals revision work. re:Work with Google. [Video file]. Retrieved from https://www.youtube.com/watch?v=C_igfnctYjA

Wrzesniewski, A., & Dutton, J. E., (2001). Crafting a job: Revisioning employees as active crafters of their work. *Academy of Management Review, 26*, 179–201.

Wrzesniewski, A., Dutton, J., & Debebe, G. (2003). Interpersonal sensemaking and the meaning of work. *Research in Organizational Behavior, 25*, 93–135.

Wrzesniewski, A., McCauley, C., Rozin, P., & Schwartz, B. (1997). Jobs, careers, and callings: People's relations to their work. *Journal of Research in Personality, 31*, 21–33.

Yeager, J. M., Fisher, S. W., & Shearon, D. N. (2011). *Smart strengths: Building character, resilience and relationships in youth*. Putnam Valley, NY: Kravis.

Index

acceptance, 46, 148
acronym, x, 157
active constructive response, 98–99, 176
administrator turnover, 113
adult school community, 93, 100, 105
adult social and emotional learning (SEL) skills, 68, 107, 128, 215. *See also* social and emotional skill set; teacher social-emotional learning (SEL)
agency thinking, 91, 136, 156, 169, 170
agility, 66, 134, 156, 157
annoyance, 64, 97
appreciation, 3, 5, 7, 18, 24, 28, 50, 53, 93, 100, 130, 135, 136, 150, 155, 156
appreciative eye, 100
attentive listening skills, 93
attitude, 25, 49, 53, 81, 93, 106, 148, 149
attrition, xvii, 142
availability, 80, 105

beginning, 8, 13, 38, 42, 46, 78, 80
belief, 3, 6, 9, 16, 18, 25, 37, 58, 62, 64, 110, 113, 132, 155, 156, 169, 171
belonging, 2, 25
benefit-finding, 134
Berlyne, Daniel, 117
best practice, 127, 130, 134–135
bias, 18, 58, 64, 132, 159, 176. *See also* confirmation bias; negativity bias; positive expectation bias
bitterness, 103

blind spot, 64, 132. *See also* blindness; change blindness; inattentional blindness
blindness, 131, 159, 175. *See also* blind spot; change blindness; inattentional blindness
boast, 88, 94
bond, 47, 76, 80, 100, 104, 104–105, 136
boredom, 122, 125
boundary, 80, 112
breaks, 123
breath, 87, 95, 143–144
budget, 103
buffer, 76, 136

calm, 72, 87, 144
celebrate, 39, 49, 81, 99, 135, 136
celebration, 20, 78, 98
(CHAMPS)^2, 157, 158
change blindness, 159, 175. *See also* blind spot; blindness; inattentional blindness
change fatigue, 90, 121, 128
chronic disconnection, 87
classroom environment, 18, 19, 68, 69, 70, 71–72, 74, 76
classroom management, 18, 30, 73, 123
collaborate, 73, 88, 93, 109, 111, 112, 120
Collaborative for Academic, Social and Emotional Learning (CASEL), 68, 77, 176, 177
community guidelines, 73

210 Index

compassion, 10, 11, 24, 63, 86, 87, 144, 156, 157. *See also* self-compassion
competency, 105
compliant, 48
conditioned reactivity, 62
confidence, 27, 46, 113, 117, 133, 142
confirmation bias, 17, 60, 61. *See also* bias
contagion, 91, 104, 107–108, 149, 171. *See also* emotional contagion
contemplative practice, 64, 144
contract, 103
contribute to the relationship, 61, 62, 63, 64, 92, 131
Cooperrider, David, 94, 100
creative, 23, 90, 103, 125, 126, 171
Cuban, Larry, 127, 154
cultural awareness, 41, 42, 74
cultural background, xv, 18, 41, 41–42, 75
cultural continuity, 70
cultural environment, 18, 19, 153. *See also* school culture
cultural proficiency, 41
culturally responsive teaching, 42
curricula, 29, 38, 48, 90, 104, 108, 119, 120–121, 123, 124, 126, 142, 143, 147, 171

dance, 27
data, 90, 102, 110, 176
David, Susan, 66, 98, 156
demoralization, 28–29, 31, 89, 90, 112
diverse, xi, 5, 39, 68, 96, 119, 168
diversity, xv, 69, 168
dull lessons, 124

educational equity, 159, 176
efficacy, 50, 88, 90, 113–114, 136, 150
effort, 3, 8, 20, 28, 47, 49, 50, 54, 62, 72, 81, 109, 113, 117, 134, 145, 147, 149
emotion, 10, 29, 55, 59, 62, 65, 66, 68, 72, 86, 98, 128, 129, 147, 149, 155, 170, 171. *See also* emotional contagion; negative emotion; positive emotion
emotional agility, 66, 134, 156
emotional contagion, 104, 107–108, 149. *See also* contagion; emotion; negative emotion; positive emotion
empathy, 10, 14
engagement, 3, 35, 47, 48, 49, 85, 93, 124

Engel, Susan, 117
equanimity, 66, 89
equitable, 18, 132
ethical, 45, 47
exemplary rating, xiii
exercise, 27, 149
expectation, 16, 17, 18, 37, 38, 39, 46, 60, 62, 71, 73, 77, 91, 107, 119, 169, 172. *See also* high expectations
experiences of teachers of color, 159, 175
experiment, 16, 33, 35, 61, 119, 122, 125, 126, 157

faculty protocols and activities, 159, 176
fault-finding, 134
filibustering, 124
Fisher, Bobbi, xii
five good things, 54
flexibility, 76, 125, 147
forgiveness, 63
Fredrickson, Barbara, 75–76, 136
fun, 54, 75, 97, 124, 125, 126, 139, 149, 177

goal, xiii, 27, 38, 39, 49, 104, 125. *See also* meaningful goals
grandparent, 25, 40–41, 141
Grant, Adam, 3
grateful, 93, 151
gratitude, 75, 76, 136, 150, 151, 156, 159, 171, 176
greet, 20, 34, 35, 48, 51, 93
group development, 75
growth fostering relationship, 54, 87
growth mindset, 50. *See also* mind-set

Hammond, Zaretta, 42, 176
Handbook of Research on Teachers of Color, xv, 175
health, 3, 30, 68, 93, 98, 103, 104, 122, 131, 140, 143, 146, 172
heart, 104, 106, 170
high expectations, 8, 9, 26, 67, 68. *See also* expectations
hospital study, 2, 3
Howells, Kerry, 148, 150
humble, 128
humility, 119, 128, 130, 153, 155, 157
humor, 75, 97, 108

identity, xv, 68, 69, 148
imperfect, 119, 145, 146, 155
implicit cognition, 159, 176
improvisation, 127, 154
inattentional blindness, 159. *See also* blind spot; blindness; change blindness
individualized education plan (IEP), 15, 140
inequities, 24
inner dialogue, 65, 170
inspiration, 75, 76, 99, 136, 149
integrity, 105, 106
intelligence, 90, 154, 171
interdependence, 85, 130
interpersonal curiosity, 37, 155
interpret, 60, 61, 64, 69, 95, 96–97, 127, 128, 167, 168
interpretation, 41, 42, 74, 75, 94, 95, 122, 154, 157, 167
interreactivity, 62
intrapersonal, 97, 126, 155
intrinsic, 49
isolation, 88

Jackson, Philip, 127
job description, 2–3
job security, 142
joy, 23, 75, 76, 98, 100, 136, 150, 151
judgment, xiii, 13, 19, 42, 45, 65, 89, 127

Kanter, Rosabeth, 120
kind, 26, 58, 69, 86, 87, 105, 145–146, 171
kindness, 9, 25, 26, 58, 75, 81, 105, 135
Kuhl, Patricia, 72

laugh, 7, 75, 108, 149, 151
less is more, 123
Levy, Steven, xii
love of learning, 50–51

make it work, 31, 59, 103, 147
mandate, 28, 90, 102, 143
meaningful goals, 91, 136, 156, 169, 170, 173
mediocrity, 8
memory, 50, 57, 72, 117, 128, 129, 133, 149
mentor, 142–143
Miller, Jean Baker, 54

Milner, H. Richard, 59
mind-set, 122, 142. *See also* growth mindset
mindful, 10, 42, 64, 86–87, 118, 140, 144, 149
mindful awareness, 64, 144, 155, 157
mindfulness, 63, 64, 64–65, 112, 142, 144, 159, 176
mistake, 14, 25, 40, 41–42, 50, 61, 86, 118, 119, 145, 155
moral commitments, 31
mortifying, 6

Neff, Kristin, 146, 177
negative emotion, 57–58, 62, 104, 134; perception, 62, 75. *See also* emotion; emotional contagion
negative talk, 92, 94, 103
negativity, 92, 93, 95, 106, 149
negativity bias, 60, 61, 108, 134, 148. *See also* bias
norm, 41, 67, 73, 74

observe, 6, 48, 79, 86, 95–96, 108, 110
one-on-one, 6, 46, 52, 73–74, 78, 135
optimism, 172
organize, 37, 70–71, 89, 140
outreach, 78

Palmer, Parker, x, xi, 148, 154
Pasteur, Louis, 139
pathway thinking, 91, 136, 156, 169, 170, 173
patience, 143–144
personal narrative, 170
personal regard, 105
perspicacity, 153–154, 158
positive emotion, 75, 104, 134, 136; perception, 62, 75, 82. *See also* emotion; emotional contagion
positive expectation bias, 172. *See also* bias
positivity, 10, 20, 50, 66, 75, 76, 134, 135, 136, 149–150, 156, 157
power to, 100
praise, 14, 109
predictable, 70, 71, 74
presupposition, 62, 119

priority, 26, 37, 54, 58, 78, 101, 107, 108, 112, 119
priorities, xvii, 37, 54, 89–90, 91, 122, 170
privileges, 167
professional development, xvi, 95, 120, 125
professional freedom, 104

qualitative research, xiii
question-answer cycle, 74

rationale, xvii, 17, 20, 23, 66, 68, 123, 128
reactivity, 62, 64, 144
receptivity, 125
recharge, 65, 80, 123
relational, 1–2, 2, 18, 33, 35, 54, 64, 75, 128, 150
relational-cultural context, 18, 67, 87, 155
relational-cultural theory (RCT), x, 87
relational interest, 37
relational trust, 99–100, 104, 105–106, 107, 136
relax, 20, 65, 143, 146
renew, 80, 91, 131, 144, 149
reputation, 14, 17, 20, 61, 81, 83, 95
resilience, 58, 76, 86, 107, 136, 150, 170
respect, 6, 14, 46, 48, 53, 58, 69, 93, 104, 105, 122, 143
respectful, 41, 53, 58, 61, 101, 129
Richmond, Geraldine, 168
risk, 27, 34, 72, 73, 118
Roediger, Roddy, 133
routine, 19, 70–71, 71, 73, 110

safe, 16, 24, 25, 34, 46, 47, 62, 71, 72, 79, 106, 113, 144
Santoro, Doris, 28–29, 31, 90, 112
savor, 50, 98, 99, 136, 143–144, 150, 151, 156, 177
school culture, 30, 107, 111. *See also* cultural environment
selective attention, 157, 159, 175
self-compassion, 86, 87, 146, 156, 177. *See also* compassion
self-criticism, 86
Seppala, Emma, 10, 86–87
sing, 27
Singer, Tania, 10

social and emotional skill set, 57, 68, 81, 89, 107. *See also* social, emotional, and cognitive; teacher social emotional learning (SEL)
social brain, 72
social, emotional, and cognitive, 101. *See also* Collaborative for Academic, Social and Emotional Learning (CASEL)
social species, 1, 45, 67, 153, 171
soul, 106, 140
staff meeting, 95, 112
standpoint theory, 167, 167–168
stereotype, 40, 75, 132
stereotypic association, 40
story line, 97, 98, 170
storytelling, 99
strength, 2, 16, 47, 51, 52, 63, 91, 100, 107, 118, 125, 140, 141, 149, 156, 157, 163, 169, 177, 178
strength-finding, 134
students' reinvention of themselves, 13
success-based habit, 118

tap in/tap out, 89
teacher social emotional learning (SEL), 68. *See also* adult social and emotional learning (SEL) skills; social and emotional skill set
teaching style, 19
technology, 78, 80, 141
thank you, 83, 109, 135
thankful, 136, 150, 156
thankless job, 5
theory of mind, 74
think on your feet, 127, 129, 154
thought-action repertoire, 75
thought-feeling awareness, 63
toxic, 103
translation, 78
two scenarios about crossing a room, 33, 35, 47

universal design for learning (UDL), 38
upward spiral, 76, 136

vent, 82, 87, 103, 148
verbal check-in, 93
verbally correcting, 6
vision, 24, 28, 71, 101, 171

well-being, ix, xi, xvii, 23, 28, 30, 54, 94, 98, 104–105, 114, 122, 131, 134, 136, 142, 144, 178
wellness, 142
whole child, 102
willpower, 58

wishing, 172

yelling, 106

zest, 54, 100

About the Author

Betsy Nordell, Ed.D., is a former classroom teacher and current teacher educator with more than 30 years of experience in a variety of educational settings. Since 1993, she has been teaching and coaching administrators and teachers with Open Circle, a Wellesley Centers for Women (WCW) Project at Wellesley College. Betsy is also a trainer and coach with Leading Together, a program out of the Center for Courage and Renewal, Northeast. She earned her BSBA in management (with minors in education and personnel selection and development) from Bucknell University. She spent seven years in the corporate sector before earning her M.Ed. from Wheelock College and her teaching and learning doctorate from American International College. Her research, publications, presentations, and workshops have focused on the creation of optimal learning communities, adult social and emotional learning, perception and bias, mindfulness, curiosity, gratitude, compassion, and hope and the power of positive relationships to foster growth.